New Developments in Medical Research

Connective Tissue

Types, Functions and Clinical Aspects

NEW DEVELOPMENTS IN MEDICAL RESEARCH

Additional books and e-books in this series can be found on Nova's website under the Series tab.

New Developments in Medical Research

Connective Tissue

Types, Functions and Clinical Aspects

Jim M. Pearson
Editor

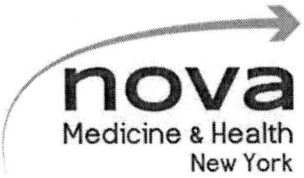

Copyright © 2020 by Nova Science Publishers, Inc.

All rights reserved. No part of this book may be reproduced, stored in a retrieval system or transmitted in any form or by any means: electronic, electrostatic, magnetic, tape, mechanical photocopying, recording or otherwise without the written permission of the Publisher.

We have partnered with Copyright Clearance Center to make it easy for you to obtain permissions to reuse content from this publication. Simply navigate to this publication's page on Nova's website and locate the "Get Permission" button below the title description. This button is linked directly to the title's permission page on copyright.com. Alternatively, you can visit copyright.com and search by title, ISBN, or ISSN.

For further questions about using the service on copyright.com, please contact:
Copyright Clearance Center
Phone: +1-(978) 750-8400 Fax: +1-(978) 750-4470 E-mail: info@copyright.com.

NOTICE TO THE READER

The Publisher has taken reasonable care in the preparation of this book, but makes no expressed or implied warranty of any kind and assumes no responsibility for any errors or omissions. No liability is assumed for incidental or consequential damages in connection with or arising out of information contained in this book. The Publisher shall not be liable for any special, consequential, or exemplary damages resulting, in whole or in part, from the readers' use of, or reliance upon, this material. Any parts of this book based on government reports are so indicated and copyright is claimed for those parts to the extent applicable to compilations of such works.

Independent verification should be sought for any data, advice or recommendations contained in this book. In addition, no responsibility is assumed by the Publisher for any injury and/or damage to persons or property arising from any methods, products, instructions, ideas or otherwise contained in this publication.

This publication is designed to provide accurate and authoritative information with regard to the subject matter covered herein. It is sold with the clear understanding that the Publisher is not engaged in rendering legal or any other professional services. If legal or any other expert assistance is required, the services of a competent person should be sought. FROM A DECLARATION OF PARTICIPANTS JOINTLY ADOPTED BY A COMMITTEE OF THE AMERICAN BAR ASSOCIATION AND A COMMITTEE OF PUBLISHERS.

Additional color graphics may be available in the e-book version of this book.

Library of Congress Cataloging-in-Publication Data

ISBN: 978-1-53617-875-3

Library of Congress Control Number: 2020937113

Published by Nova Science Publishers, Inc. † New York

CONTENTS

Preface vii

Chapter 1 Periodontal Connective Tissue: An Update 1
*Nikesh N. Moolya, Nilima Rajhans,
Shraddha Mali, Samkhya AP,
Bhagyashree Bhargude and Pratibha Shirsath*

Chapter 2 Connective Tissue Graft 93
Shruti Bhatnagar

Chapter 3 Subepithelial Connective Tissue
Grafts (SCTGs) in Periodontology 113
Aysan Lektemur Alpan and Nebi Cansin Karakan

Index 141

PREFACE

The human body is composed of four basic kinds of tissue: nervous, muscular, epithelial, and connective tissue. Connective tissue is the most abundant type and serves as a connecting link for binding, supporting and strengthening all other body tissues.

In this compilation, the authors explore connective tissue grafts, a promising and reliable method that provides a satisfactory esthetic outcome, making it a popular option for clinicians.

The fundamentals of subepithelial connective tissue grafts, harvesting techniques, clinical success and possible postoperative complications is also discussed.

Chapter 1 - The human body is composed of four basic kinds of tissue: nervous, muscular, epithelial, and connective tissue. Connective tissue is the most abundant, widely distributed, varied type and serves as a connecting link for binding, supporting and strengthening all other body tissues together. It includes fibrous tissues, fat, cartilage, bone, bone marrow, and blood. It is distinguished from the other types in that the matrix usually occupies more space than the cells do, and the cells are relatively far apart. The matrix of connective tissue typically consists of fibers and a featureless ground substance. The most abundant fiber in connective tissues is a protein called collagen. Collagen, as is leather, consists of the connective tissue layer (dermis) of animal skins. Collagen also strengthens bone and cartilage. Elastic and reticular fibers are less abundant connective tissue proteins with a more limited distribution. Some of the cells of connective tissue are fibroblasts (which produce collagen fibers and are the only cell type in tendons and ligaments); adipocytes (fat cells); leukocytes (white blood cells, also found outside the bloodstream in fibrous connective tissues); macrophages (large phagocytic cells descended from certain leukocytes); erythrocytes (red blood cells, found only in the blood and bone marrow); chondrocytes (cartilage cells); and osteocytes (bone cells). The oral cavity is lined by a mucous membrane that consists of two layers: epithelial and connective tissue (lamina propria). Histologically the oral mucosa can be classified as masticatory, lining and specialized mucosa. The masticatory mucosa is made up of gingiva and hard palate. The characteristic features of the gingiva are determined by inherent factors in the tissue rather than being the result of functional adaptation and that the differentiation (keratinization) of the gingival epithelium is controlled by morphogenetic stimuli from the underlying connective tissue. This chapter aims to assess the role of connective tissue along with emphasis on clinical aspects. Conclusion: Connective tissue components allow for the interaction of the teeth with external forces and helps prevent damage in function. Knowing the structure and origin of the components that constitute the connective tissue, the interaction with each other and their biological and physical limits is crucial if one has to understand the changes seen in the connective when affected by disease and excessive occlusal forces.

Chapter 2 - Connective tissue graft is a promising and reliable method that provides a satisfactory esthetic outcome, making it a popular alternative for clinicians. It can be described as a free autogenous graft. The surgical procedure was first described by Alan Edel in 1974 for increase in width of attached gingiva. It is generally used to obtain root coverage following gingival recession, which was a later development by Burt Langer in the early 1980s. The SCTG is obtained usually from the palatal area, tuberosity area, retromolar pad area too. The advantages of the SCTG are that it is inexpensive, versatile, and easily available; it provides successful outcomes; it is less invasive than other autogenous harvesting techniques; and it has a shorter healing period. Apart from this SCTG also have osteogenic, chondrogenic and mesenchymal properties. A connective tissue graft also could be used as a barrier for furcation defects and intrabony defects.

Chapter 3 - Periodontal plastic surgery applications have increased in modern dentistry as the importance of patients to their appearance. For this purpose, many techniques and flap designs have been used to treat gingival recession, but subepithelial connective tissue graft (SCTG) seems to be the gold standard procedure. SCTGs can be harvested from several areas in the mouth such as maxillary tuberosity and palate with different approaches which can affect graft quality and postoperative complications. In this section, rationale of SCTG, harvesting techniques, clinical success and possible postoperative complications will be discussed in the light of literature.

In: Connective Tissue
Editor: Jim M. Pearson

ISBN: 978-1-53617-875-3
© 2020 Nova Science Publishers, Inc.

Chapter 1

PERIODONTAL CONNECTIVE TISSUE: AN UPDATE

Nikesh N. Moolya, Nilima Rajhans, PhD, Shraddha Mali, Samkhya AP, Bhagyashree Bhargude and Pratibha Shirsath

Department of Periodontology, YCMM and RDF Dental College, Ahmednagar, Maharashtra, India

ABSTRACT

The human body is composed of four basic kinds of tissue: nervous, muscular, epithelial, and connective tissue. Connective tissue is the most abundant, widely distributed, varied type and serves as a connecting link for binding, supporting and strengthening all other body tissues together. It includes fibrous tissues, fat, cartilage, bone, bone marrow, and blood. It is distinguished from the other types in that the matrix usually occupies more space than the cells do, and the cells are relatively far apart. The matrix of connective tissue typically consists of fibers and a featureless ground substance. The most abundant fiber in connective tissues is a protein called collagen. Collagen, as is leather, consists of the connective tissue layer (dermis) of animal skins. Collagen also strengthens bone and cartilage. Elastic and reticular fibers are less abundant connective tissue proteins with a more limited distribution. Some of the cells of connective tissue are fibroblasts (which produce collagen fibers and are the only cell type in tendons and ligaments); adipocytes (fat cells); leukocytes (white blood cells, also found outside the bloodstream in fibrous connective tissues); macrophages (large phagocytic cells descended from certain leukocytes); erythrocytes (red blood cells, found only in the blood and bone marrow); chondrocytes (cartilage cells); and osteocytes (bone cells).

The oral cavity is lined by a mucous membrane that consists of two layers: epithelial and connective tissue (lamina propria). Histologically the oral mucosa can be classified as masticatory, lining and specialized mucosa. The masticatory mucosa is made up of gingiva and hard palate. The characteristic features of the gingiva are determined by inherent factors in the tissue rather than being the result of functional adaptation and that the differentiation (keratinization) of the gingival epithelium is controlled by morphogenetic stimuli from the underlying connective tissue. This chapter aims to assess the role of connective tissue along with emphasis on clinical aspects.

Conclusion: Connective tissue components allow for the interaction of the teeth with external forces and helps prevent damage in function. Knowing the structure and origin of the components that constitute the connective tissue, the interaction with each other and their biological and physical limits is crucial if one has to understand the changes seen in the connective when affected by disease and excessive occlusal forces.

INTRODUCTION

"I am less interested in skin than in fascia." - Mathew Barney

Life is a sequence of complex molecules: In the connective tissue there are polymers and the most abundant protein polymer in existence. Johannes Peter Müller coined the word "connective tissue" (in German, Bindegewebe) in 1830. The tissue was already known in the 18th century as a distinct group. This arises from the mesenchyme, which is the middle layer of three embryonic germ layers (Bancroft JD, Gamble M,). The term connect comes from the Latin word 'connecture,' which means' to bind' (Frank, Khan and Hashmi 2004). This type of tissue does much more than simply connecting structures. It can do wrapping, filling and packaging as well as serving as a soft buffer between structures as well as form strong supporting structures such as bones. The human body is not simply a set of separate parts but a cohesive network of tissues. It covers, assists and penetrates all the muscles, bones, nerves and organs. It forms and gives its strength to the human body. Connective tissue is present everywhere in the body, including the nervous system and between other tissues. The three external membranes (meninges) that surround the brain and spinal cord are made up of connective tissue in the central nervous system.

Connective tissue comprises three main components: fibers (elastic and collagen fibers), ground substance and cells like fibroblasts, adipocytes, macrophages, mast cells and leucocytes. In contrast to epithelia, connective tissue contains few cells and an extensive extracellular matrix comprising protein fibers, glycoproteins, and proteoglycans. It may serve as a medium of contact between other tissues and cells and plays an important role in the body's defense mechanisms. The role of this tissue is to provide structural and mechanical support for other tissues and to mediate the exchange between the circulation and other tissues of nutrients and waste. There are two main components in these tissues, an extracellular matrix and several support cells. Most often, their quality of three distinct types of extracellular fibers define the different connective tissues: collagenous fibers, elastic fibers, and reticular fibers.

CELLS OF CONNECTIVE TISSUE

Depending on their location and type of organ or structure, different types of cells are present in connective tissue, such as fibroblast, myofibroblast, adipose cells, mast cells, tissue macrophages, white blood cells, osteoblast, chondroblast, and cells forming blood (Ross 1975, Dorfman 1959). Usually, the intercellular substance consists of both amorphous (non-sulphated and sulphated mucopolysaccharides), collagen, reticular and elastic fibers formed elements. The intercellular ground substance's function is to form the matrix by which metabolites are transported. Non-cellular material covers the cellular substance. The cell-to-cell ratio ranges from one type of connective tissue to another.

Connective tissue exists with various physical properties in many different forms. It can be broadly categorized into normal connective tissue and special connective tissue. The proper connective tissue consists of loose connective tissue and dense connective tissue (which is further subdivided into dense regular and dense irregular connective tissue). Loose and dense connective tissue is distinguished by the ratio of ground to fibrous tissue. Loose connective tissue has a much greater ground material and a relative lack of fibrous tissue, while dense connective tissue is the opposite. Dense normal connective tissue, found in structures such as tendons and ligaments, is characterized by collagen fibers organized in an ordered parallel manner, giving it one-way tensile strength with its dense bundles of fibers arranged in all directions; dense irregular connective tissue provides strength in multiple directions.

Mesenchyme is a type of connective tissue present in the development of embryo organs that can differentiate between all forms of mature connective tissue. The mucous connective tissue known as Wharton's jelly, found inside the umbilical cord, is another form of fairly undifferentiated connective tissue (Troyer and Weiss 2008).

Different types of different tissues and cells are categorized within the connective tissue continuum and are as diverse as brown and white adipose tissue, hair, cartilage and bone. Certain types of connective tissues include tissues that are fibrous, elastic and lymphoid. Fibroareolar tissue is a mix of fibrous and areolar tissue. Fibromuscular tissue consists of muscle and fibrous tissue. In the process of wound healing, new vascularized connective tissue is called granulation tissue. Immune system cells such as macrophages, mast cells, plasma cells, and eosinophils are found dispersed in loose connective tissue, providing the ground for antigen detection to cause inflammatory and immune responses.

Adipocytes (Fat cells) (Hassan, Latif, and Yacoub 2012)

Adipocytes appear like a signet-ring that stores lipid and act as an empty space. They're not separated into pieces but may occur in loose areolar tissue, or as in adipose tissue, they may occur in clusters. Within adipocytes, lipids are present. A lipid is generally regarded as an organic substance insoluble in water, soluble in organic solvents or partly soluble in water. Lipids are usually found as a portion of all tissues in the form of stored lipids or lipid structures like myelin. These may be protein-bound (lipoprotein) or carbohydrates (glycolipids) (Figure 1)

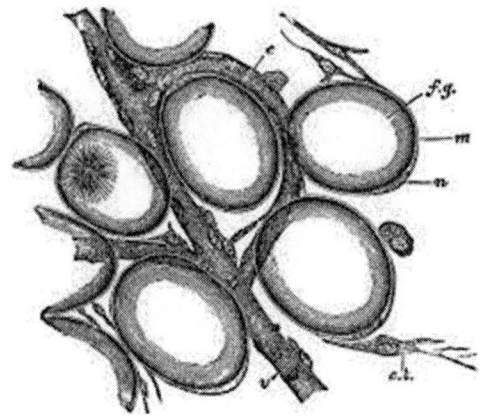

Figure 1. Adipose cells.

Mesenchymal Cells (Bhartiya 2013)

Mesenchymal cells are undifferentiated cells that have a stellate cytoplasm. These are pluripotent cells that run along blood vessels Macrophages (Histiocytes) Free and Fixed type Fixed Cells (histiocytes)- These are irregular shaped short branching processes with dark indented eccentric nucleus, derived from monocyte involved in phagocytosis and fused to form giant cells. The macrophage is the connective tissue representing the system of the reticuloendothelial, or mononuclear phagocyte. This system comprises a variety of tissue-specific, mobile, phagocytic cells originating from monocytes-including the liver's Kupffer cells, the lung's alveolar macrophages, the central nervous system's microglia and spleen's reticular cells. Macrophages are distinct from fibroblasts, but can be detected when large amounts of visible tracer substances such as coloring or carbon particles are internalized. In the connective tissue surface, macrophages phagocytose foreign material and also play an important role as a cell presenting antigen. (Figure 2)

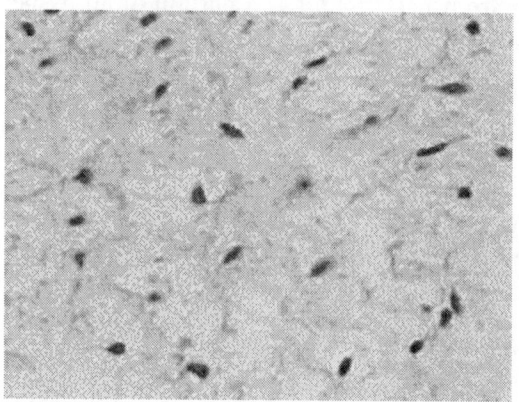

Figure 2. Mesenchymal cells.

Mast Cells (da Silva, Jamur, and Oliver 2014)

Mast cell is thought to be a phylogenetically ancient cell that tends to occur with blood circulation in all animals. Human mast cells usually appear as round or elongated cells with a diameter ranging from 8-20 micrometers under a light microscope. Mast cells release various substances such as histamine as well as various types of enzymes and factors. Histamine release is associated with allergic reaction production when a tissue is exposed to a susceptible antigen. Although more than a century ago, mast cells were discovered, their functions go beyond their role in allergic reactions and remain elusive until recently. However, there is a growing appreciation that the recognition of pathogens and modulation of appropriate immune responses are an important physiological function of these cells. Mast cells were shown to be crucial for optimal immune responses during infection due to their ability to instantly release several pro-inflammatory mediators from intracellular stores and their location at the host-environment interface. Mast cells are typically found in connective tissue granulated cells. The immune responses to foreign particles are regulated by these cells. In particular, in response to antigen recognition, they release large amounts of histamine and enzymes. This cycle of degranulation is protective when foreign organisms invade the body, but is also the cause of many allergic reactions. (Figure 3)

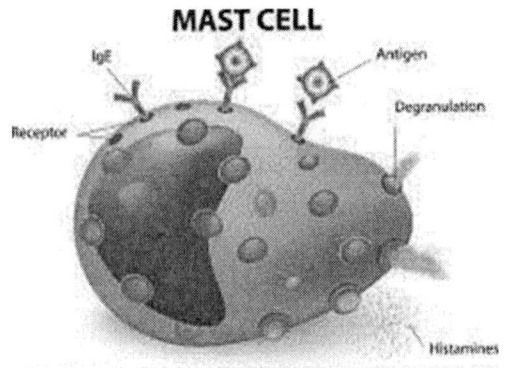

Figure 3. Mast cell.

Plasma Cells (JF. 1986)

Plasma cells are massive lymphocytes with an excess of cytoplasm and a distinctive light microscopy appearance. In a typical cartwheel or clock face configuration, they have basophilic cytoplasm and an eccentric nucleus of heterochromatin. A cytoplasm also contains a pale area containing a large Golgi apparatus and centrioles on electron microscopy. Combined with a well-developed Golgi system, abundant rough endoplasmic reticulum renders plasma cells ideal for immunoglobulin secretion. Other organelles include ribosomes, lysosomes, mitochondria, and plasma membrane in a blood cell. (Figure 4)

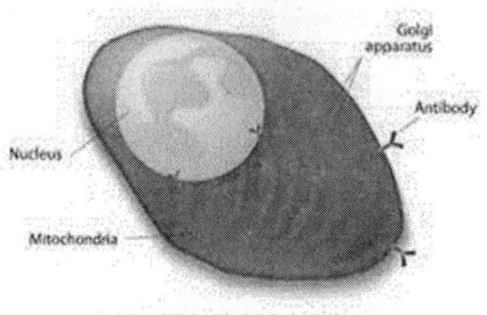

Figure 4. Plasma cell.

Cartilage (Alberts B, Johnson A, Lewis J, Raff M, Roberts K, 2002)

Cartilage is a specialized type of connective tissue formed by chondrocytes called differentiated fibroblast-like cells. A prominent extracellular matrix consisting of different proportions of connective tissue fibers embedded in a gel-like matrix characterizes it. In the matrix, they develop around themselves and chondrocytes are located within lacunae. Individual lacunae can contain multiple progenitor-derived cells. Lacunae are isolated from each other because of the chondrocyte's secretory activity. A highly fibrous, ordered, dense connective tissue capsule known as the cartilage covers the perichondrium. This layer's fibroblast-like cells have chondrogenic potential and are responsible for expanding cartilage plates through appositional development. Appositional development requires cell division, differentiation, and secretion of new extracellular matrix, thereby adding mass and new cells on the surface of the cartilage. It contrasts with interstitial growth, which deposits new matrix within mature cartilage.

Three types of cartilage are classified by the abundance of certain fibers and their matrix characteristics:

- *Hyaline cartilage* (Alberts B, Johnson A, Lewis J, Raff M, Roberts K 2002) has a matrix made up of collagen type II and chondromucoprotein, a protein-based copolymer of chondroitin sulfates A and C. It appears intensely basophilic under H&E due to its high concentration of negatively charged sulfate groups. This cartilage is located in the nose, the tracheal rings, and the sternum is joined by the ribs.
- *Fibrocartilage* is distinguished by its high content and orderly arrangement of type I collagen fibers. It is usually located in areas where ribs, intervertebral disks, and pubic symphysis are connected to tendons.
- *Elastic cartilage* (Alberts B, Johnson A, Lewis J, Raff M, Roberts K 2002) has an abundance of elastic fibers and is quite cellular. This consists of collagen type II and is found in the ear auricle and the epiglottis.

Connective tissue has a wide range of functions depending on the cell types and the various fiber groups involved. Loose and dense irregular connective tissue, produced mainly by fibroblasts and collagen fibers, play an important role in providing a medium for oxygen and nutrients to pass from capillaries to cells, as well as carbon dioxide and waste materials to flow back into circulation from cells. These also allow organs to withstand forces that stretch and tear. Dense regular connective tissue, which forms organized structures, is a major functional component of tendons, ligaments and aponeurosis, and is also found in highly specialized organs such as cornea (Parry DA 1984). Made of elastin and fibrillin, elastic fibers also provide resistance to stretch forces. They are found in large blood vessel walls and in certain ligaments, particularly in the ligamenta flava. (Figure 5)

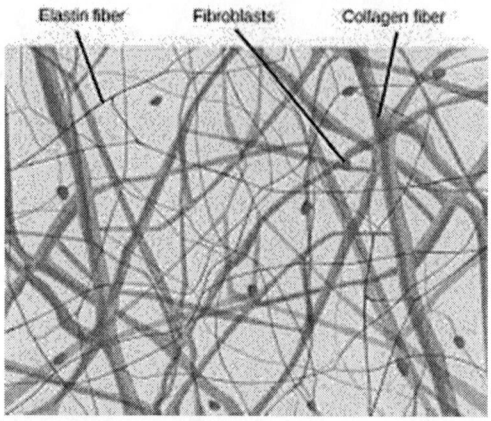

Figure 5. Fibers of connective tissue.

Reticular fibers made by reticular cells provide the stroma or structural support for the parenchyma or functional portion of the body in hematopoietic and lymphatic tissues. Not every form of CT is fibrous. Adipose tissue and blood are sources of non-fibrous CT. Among other functions, adipose tissue gives the body "mechanical cushioning." Although there is no large collagen network in adipose tissue, collagen fibers and collagen sheets hold groups of adipose cells together to keep fat tissue under pressure (for instance, foot sole). The blood matrix is plasma.

Collagenous Fibers (Ushiki 2002)

Collagenous fibers comprise collagen types I, II, or III and are present in all connective tissue types. Based on the ratio of collagen fibers to ground substance, collagenous connective tissue is divided into two types. The most abundant form of collagenous connective tissue is the loose areolar connective tissue. It takes place in thin, elongated bundles separated by regions containing ground material. Dense connective tissue is enriched with a small ground substance in collagen fibers. If the closely packed fibers bundles are in one direction, they are called regular; if they are oriented in multiple directions, they are referred to as irregular. An example of normal dense connective tissue is tendon tissue; the dermis is an example of irregular dense connective tissue.

Reticular Fibers

Reticular fibers comprise collagen type III. Unlike the collagenous fibers that are dense and coarse, reticular fibers form a thin reticular network. This network is widespread across multiple tissues and form supporting structures in the liver, lymphoid organs, capillary endothelia, and muscle fibers.

Elastic Fibers

Elastic fibers contain the elastin protein that co-polymerizes with the fibrillin protein. As in the walls of arteries, these fibers are often organized into lamellar plates. The ligaments are characterized by dense, regular, elastic tissue. Elastic fibers can be extended because they are usually disorganized–stretching them helps them take on an ordered form.

Ground Substance

The ground substance is an aqueous gel of glycoproteins and proteoglycans that occupies the space between the connective tissue's cellular and fibrillary elements. A gel-like viscous consistency characterizes it and is polyanionic. The ground substance's characteristics dictate the permeability to solutes and proteins of the connective tissue layer. The CT matrix is formed by both the ground substance and the proteins (fibers). The mesenchyme comes from the connective tissue. Loose connective tissue in most organs acts as a biological packing material with more specific functions between cells and other tissues.

Dense connective tissue form provides the skin's dermis with hard physical support

Desmoulière, Guyot, and Gabbiani (2004) reviewed and discussed the mechanism of myofibroblast evolution during fibrotic and malignant conditions and the interaction of myofibroblasts with other cells in order to control tumor progression. On this basis they suggested that the myofibroblast may represent a new important target of antitumor therapy.

Boris Hinz (2007) observed specific molecular features as well as factors that control myofibroblast differentiation are potential targets to counteract its development, function, and survival. Such targets include a-smooth muscle actin and more recently discovered markers of the myofibroblast cytoskeleton, membrane surface proteins, and the extracellular matrix.

Olivier De Wever et al. (2008) found that myofibroblasts and cancer associated fibroblasts are important components of the tumor stroma. The origin of myofibroblasts remains controversial, although fibroblasts and bone marrow-derived precursors are considered to be the main progenitor cells. Myofibroblast reactions also occur in fibrosis. Therefore, we wonder whether non tumorous myofibroblasts have different characteristics and different origins as compared to tumor associated myofibroblasts.

Eliene-Magda de-Assis et al. (2011) evaluated the presence of stromal myofibroblasts in oral lichen planus and oral squamous cell carcinoma, They observed that the presence of stromal myofibroblasts were present as negative in 11 (26.8%), scanty in 15 (36.6%), and abundant in 15 samples (36.6%). The presence of stromal myofibroblasts was statistically higher in high-invasive oral squamous cell carcinoma than in low invasive oral squamous cell carcinoma.

PERIODONTAL CONNECTIVE TISSUE

The periodontium is a unique organ which comprises two soft connective tissues (gingiva and periodontal ligament) and two calcified components (cementum and alveolar bone). Because of this particular composition, the periodontium is an intriguing tissue to study with respect to its reparative and regenerative capacity. The inflammatory and fibrotic diseases affect its matrix components thus severely compromising structure and function of the periodontium. Periodontitis is one of the most common chronic inflammatory diseases affecting humans which, if left untreated and continues to progress, may result in tooth loss. The biochemistry of normal periodontal connective tissues and how they are affected by pathological conditions were reviewed previously in 1983 (Narayanan, A. S. and Page R). Since then many new collagen types and matrix proteins have been identified and the ultrastructural distribution of some of these molecules in the periodontium has been determined. More importantly, regeneration of periodontal connective tissues destroyed by inflammatory diseases has become a focus of active research as it is a major challenge to achieve a predictable outcome.

Components of the Periodontal Connective Tissue

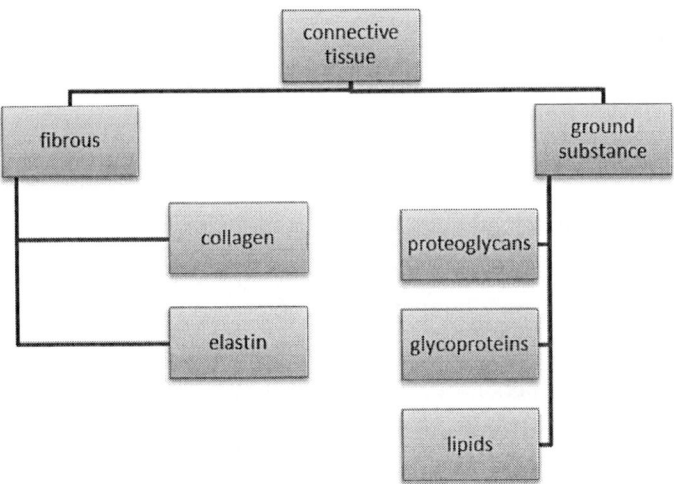

Figure 6. Components of connective tissue.

Of these components, the collagen and proteoglycans have been reasonably well characterized (Narayan AS, Bartold PM. 1987).

Collagen is a major constituent of a variety of skeletal and soft connective tissues. It has been estimated that 30 per cent of the total protein in the human body is collagen (Nimni M. 1980). These fibrous proteins are responsible principally for the maintenance of the framework and tone of the tissues. To date, eleven different types of collagen have been identified on the basis of their molecular composition (Miller EJ 1987).

Various tissues have differences in type, size, distribution and alignment of the collagen fibers and this is related to the different physical and functional properties of the tissues. The periodontium is no exception in which differences in type and quantity vary depending upon the location.

Distribution of major matrix components of the periodontium is as follows:

Site	Collagens	Proteoglycans
Gingiva	I*, III*, IV, V	HA, HS, DS*, CS
Periodontal ligament	I, III*, V	HA, HS, DS*, CS
Alveolar bone	I*	HA, HS, DS, CS*
Cementum	I, III	HA, HS, DS, CS*

Abbreviations: HA (hyaluronate); HS (heparan sulphate); DS (dermatan sulphate); CS (chondroitin sulphate).
*Indicates the predominant species present at specific site.

Electron microscopic and immunohistochemical studies have shown that the collagenous components of the periodontium are organized into distinct and discrete architectural patterns. As for most connective tissues, the fibers of the periodontium contain a heterotypic mixture of collagens of which type I is the major constituent (Narayanan, A. S. Page 1983). In the gingiva, collagen fibers are arranged either as large, dense bundles, or in a loose pattern of short thin fibers mixed with a fine reticular network and are composed primarily of both type I and type III collagen (Chavrier, C., Couble, M. L., Magloire, H. and Griniaud 1984). Several other collagenhave been identified and include types IV, V, VI, XII, and XIV. While Type I collagen has a generalized distribution throughout the lamina propria, Type III collagen has a diffuse distribution and is preferentially localized as thinner fibers with a reticular pattern near the connective tissue- epithelial interface (Narayanan, A. S., Clagett, J. A. and Page 1985). In contrast, type V collagen has a parallel filamentous pattern and appears to coat the dense fibers composed of type I and III collagen (Narayanan, A. S., Clagett, J. A. and Page 1985) (Romanos, G., Schrter-Kermani, C., Hinz, N. and Bemimoulin and P. 1991). Type VI collagen is present in the gingival connective tissue in a diffuse microfibrillar pattern,and is present near basement membranes in the rat, but not in marmoset (Romanos, G., Schrter-Kermani, C., Hinz, N. and Bemimoulin and P. 1991) In gingiva, basement membrane is present at junctions of connective tissue with epithelium and cementum, in rete pegs, as well as around blood vessels and nerves, and contains type IV collagen, laminin and heparan sulfate proteoglycan (Romanos, G., Schrter-Kermani, C., Hinz, N. and Bemimoulin and P. 1991). Presence of type IV collagen in the rat appears to be restricted to external basal lamina, while both external and internal laminae contain laminin (Sawada, T., Yamamoto, T., Yanagisawa, T., Takuma and Hasegawa, H. and Watanabe 1990).

The major ground substance in the periodontal connective tissue comprises proteoglycans and glycosaminoglycans. In the gingival connective tissue the major glycosaminoglycan (GAG) is dermatan sulfate, while heparan sulfate is the predominant GAG in the epithelium. Apart from differences in sulfation and charge, gingival GAGs manifest heterogeneity in their molecular size ranging from 15 kDa for heparan sulfate to 340 kDa for hyaluronan (Bartold 1987). To date, decorin, biglycan and versican proteoglycans have been identified in biochemical extracts of gingival tissues using antibodies and cDNA probes (Larjava, H., HWinen, L. and Rahemtulla 1992). Within the gingival tissues, dermatan sulfate appears to be associated with collagen fibers and it is prevalent at the epithelial connective tissue interface while heparan sulfate is found primarily in basement membranes of epithelium and capillary endothelium (Erlinger, R., Willerhausen-Zonnchen, B. and Welsch 1995) (Shibutani, T., Muruhashi, Y. and Iwayama 1989). Using a variety of antibodies, decorin, biglycan, versican, syndecan, CD-44 and perlecan have been identified within gingival tissues."

Decorin is closely associated with bundles of collagen fibers, especially in the subepithelial region, while biglycan, which is a relatively minor constituent of gingiva, is found in filament-like structures in the matrix near the oral epithelium (Bartold P. M. 1992).

Fibronectin is widely distributed in the gingival connective tissue and is localized over collagen fiber (Pitaru, S., Aubin, J. E., Bhargava, U. and Melcher 1987) Gingiva also contains osteonectin, vitronectin and elastin. Elastin is a minor component of the gingival connective tissues but is more abundant in the connective tissue of the more moveable and flexible adjacent alveolar mucosa (Chavrier 1990). Gingiva also contains tenascin which is present diffusely in the connective tissue and prominently near subepithelial basement membrane in the upper connective tissue and capillary blood vessels (Becker, J., Schuppan, D. and Muller 1993). Integrins are cell surface receptors for matrix proteins and several molecular species have been identified in the gingiva. These include $\beta 1$, $\beta 4$ and *a6* subunits in the cells of epithelium and basal lamina and $\alpha 1$, $\alpha 2$, $\alpha 5$, αv, and $\beta 3$ in fibroblasts (Larjava, H., Zhou, C., Larjava, 1. and Rahemtulla 1992). The latter presumably serve as receptors for collagens, fibronectin and vitronectin. In the periodontal ligament, type I is the major collagen present which also constitutes the fibrous component of the endosteal spaces of alveolar bone.

Molecular Interactions of the Connective Tissues

Although it is important to recognize the individual components of the extracellular matrix, it is essential to remember that they do not exist in isolation. Rather, they are capable of interacting with each other to contribute to the formation and organization of a comprehensive network forming the tissues in question. To date, molecular interactions between proteoglycans and collagen (Scott J. E. 1988).

Proteoglycans and hyaluronate," proteoglycans and other glycoproteins (for example, fibronectin and laminin) as well as between different proteoglycan species have been reported (LA. 1976). It is believed that such interactions result in a stabilizing effect allowing the matrix to assemble as a single functional unit. In addition to macromolecular interactions, components of the extracellular matrix can interact on the surface of cells. Cell surface associated proteoglycans and glycoproteins may act as receptors for intercellular communication and location. In addition, they may act as adhesive receptors or mediators. For example, heparan sulfate proteoglycan plays a direct role in forming adhesive bonds between plasma fibronectin while hyaluronate and chondroitin sulfate proteoglycan facilitate cell detachment and locomotion (Culp LA, Laterra J, Lark MW, Beyth RJ 1986). Another important function of extracellular components with respect to the periodontium is in relation to calcification. Although this process is still poorly understood, a role for proteoglycans similar to those isolated from cementum and alveolar bone has been proposed for the calcification of growth plate cartilage (Ponle AR 1987).

Effects of Medications on the Periodontal Connective Tissue

Regardless of the development of the above tests, one of the greatest aids in assessing periodontal status will still be an accurate compilation of the medical history of our patients. Indeed, although the development of new treatment regimes and diagnostic tests based upon biological principles is an exciting development, another area which will become increasingly relevant in the field of periodontics is that of medication-related periodontal response. The dentist must be cognizant of the fact that any agent which has the ability to alter fundamental host responses can potentially cause side effects at sites unrelated to the organ being targeted. Due to their high metabolic activity and susceptibility to acute and chronic inflammation the connective tissues of the periodontium are likely targets for the manifestation of many drug-related effects.

Hormonal Effects

A close correlation between normal physiological changes in the sex hormone levels and periodontal changes has been well documented. For example, gingivitis is a frequent finding during puberty and pregnancy (Adams D, Carney JS 1973). Indeed, the potential for the sex steroids to exert potent effects on the gingival tissues is high since gingival fibroblasts possess receptors for testosterones (Southern AL, Rapport SC 1978) and estrogen (Vittek J, Hernandez MR, Wenk EJ, Rappapon SC and AL. 1982). In addition, the sex hormones are actively metabolized in gingival tissues with chronically inflamed gingiva accumulating greater amounts of progesterone and androgen metabolites compared with normal gingiva (ElAttar TMA 1974) (Vittek J, Rapport SC, Gordon GC, Munangi PR and AL. 1979). These agents have been shown to affect the cellularity, vascularity, as well as the collagen and proteoglycan content of connective tissues significantly (Lindhe J, Branemark P-I 1967) (Kofoed JA, Houssay AB, Curbelo HM, Tocci AA and CH. 1973) (Nyman S. 1971). In addition to changing the make-up of the extracellular matrix, the sex hormones can be effectively utilized as growth factors by several of the putative periodontal pathogen (Kornman KS 1980,1982). The steroid hormones of the adrenal cortex also may be correlated with changes in the periodontium. Their adverse effects on connective tissues are decreased fibroblast proliferation, as well as altered collagen and proteoglycan synthesis (Bartold PM 1984). It is, therefore, not surprising to find that both the sex and adrenal hormones significantly affect wound healing (Nyman S. 1971). The effects of various hormones are not restricted to the soft connective tissues of the periodontium. For example, osteoporosis of the jaws, retarded formation of the periodontal bone and reduction in cementum formation have been recognized as being associated with altered levels of sex and adrenal hormones for a long time (Glickman I 1960). Although other hormones such as insulin, thyroid hormones and pituatory hormones also produce changes in connective tissues, prescription of these as medications is usually restricted to specific medical problems and they are not as widely prescribed as the steroid hormones. However, the prescription of steroids and their analogues is very prevalent in western society for a wide range of treatments (for example, oral contraceptives, osteoporosis, menopausal therapy, as well as anti-inflammatory agents), and therefore the possibility of side effects from these medications manifesting in the periodontium is high. These may range from mild gingivitis and stomatitis to 'pregnancy' epulis and granuloma formation as well as gingival overgrowth.

Gingival Overgrowth

This is frequently reported as a side effect of many medications commonly prescribed. Of these, phenytoin has been the most widely recognized and studied (Hassell T. M. 1981). The effects of this drug on connective tissue metabolism are well documented. It has been suggested that phenytoin can selectively allow a subpopulation of gingival fibroblasts to proliferate which are capable of high protein and collagen metabolism (Hassell TM, Page RC, Narayaran AS 1976). This may lead to uncontrolled deposition of extracellular matrix and resultant tissue overgrowth. Until recently, phenytoin was the only well recognized agent associated with causing gingival overgrowth. However, in the last ten years there has been an 'explosion' of agents reported in the literature to have similar effects in relation to gingival overgrowth (ElAttar TMA 1974) (Banold I'M. 1989). However, it is very likely that with the development of new drugs, further addition will be necessary. Despite the experimental observations of altered fibroblast function associated with phenytoin and cyclosporin gingival overgrowth, the fact that not all patients taking these medications develop gingival overgrowth, and that the lesions are usually confined to particular areas of the mouth, indicates that additional, unrecognized factors are involved. From several reports it seems that a crucial factor in the development of gingival overgrowth is the presence of dental plaque, since most lesions are reversible upon restoration of adequate plaque control (Banold I'M. 1989) (Deliliers GL, Santoro F, Polli N, Bohte E and E. 1986) (Rostock MH, Fry HR 1986). This being the case, it is interesting to note a similarity between plaque-induced gingival overgrowth and drug-induced gingival overgrowth. One of the presumed pathogenic components of plaque, bacterial lipopolysaccharide, is capable of altering cell membrane permeability to ions. Thus, whether the drugs which induce gingival overgrowth act to exacerbate localized plaque-induced gingival overgrowth needs to be assessed.

Non-Steroidal Anti-inflammatory Drugs (NSAIDS)

Non-steroidal anti-inflammatory drugs (NSAIDS) are agents which have potent anti-inflammatory and analgesic properties. They are commonly prescribed for patients with long-standing chronic inflammatory osteoarthritis) as well as for postoperative pain control. More recently, the use of NSAIDs in the treatment of chronic inflammatory periodontal diseases has been advocated (Williams RC, Jeffcoat MK, Kaplan ML 1985). However, as will be evident below, their use in these circumstances should be with caution due to their ability to adversely affect connective tissues. The propensity of NSAIDs to cause ulceration of the gastrointestinal tract (stomach, duodenum, and esophagus) is well known (Hart FD.). Therefore, it is not surprising that the oral cavity (which is also part of the gastrointestinal tract) also manifests complications - these may be as glossitis, stomatitis or tongue ulcerations. The NSAIDs dramatically alter not only inflammatory cell function but also influence mesenchymal cell function by disturbing the metabolism of collagen, proteoglycans and other structural proteins (KD 1987). Thus, the potential for NSAIDs to cause compromised tissue status exists and this may lead to poor resistance to chemical and mechanical abuse common of the gingival tissues. Given the ever-increasing wide prescription of these drugs, as well as an expected number of similar new products entering the market, it can be predicted that the number of patients presenting with NSAID-related gingival problems will become increasingly prevalent.

COLLAGEN

Collagen is a major structural protein in connective tissue and most abundant protein in the body, comprising about 25-30% of the total weight of proteins in the body. The fibers made up of collagen have high tensile strength. This protein is an important structural component in tissue such as periodontal ligament, and tendon in which mechanical force need to be transmitted without loss. It is the major fibrous element of tissue like bone, cartilage, tendon, teeth, blood vessel etc. Collagen transforms longitudinal tensional force into lateral comprehensive force. Apart from their structural role collagen can also influence cell shape, cell differentiation, cell proliferation, adhesion, migration and many other cellular activities. Thus it is an important multifactorial connective tissue protein that participates in many biological functions. About 72% of it is found in skin only (Sandhu, Gupta, and Singla 2012).

Functions of Collagen

1. Acts as a scaffold for our bodies.
2. Controls cell shape and differentiation.
3. Helps broken bones to regenerate and wounds to heal.
4. Helps blood vessels to grow to feed healing areas.

Structure

The triple helical structure that is known to be correct in the essentials was proposed by G. N. Ramachandran and Gopinath Kartha in the year 1954. This proposed structure came to be known as "Madras helix" (Sasisekharan and Yathindra 1999).

ELECTRON MICROSCOPIC STRUCTURE

Primary Structure

The presence of a triple helical structure formed by three polypeptide chains is called α chains (Kielty and Grant 2003). The α chains are left-handed helices, which wrap around each other into a right-handed, rope like triple helical rod. Depending on the type of collagen, the molecule may be made up of either three identical α chains, or two or three different α chains. The triple helix may be a continuous stretch, or it may be interrupted by non-collagenous segments. A special amino acid sequence makes the tight collagen triple helix, stable. Every third amino acid is a glycine, and many of the remaining amino acids are proline or hydroxyproline (Gly-X-Y). The glycine forms a tiny elbow packed inside the helix, and the proline and hydroxyproline smoothly bend the chain back around the helix. Glycine is essential for the triple-helical conformation because larger amino acids will not fit in the center of the triple helix. The top half is very uniform, where the sequence is the ideal mixture of glycine and prolines. At the bottom, the helix is less regular, because many different amino acids are placed between the equally-spaced glycines. The collagen molecule is stabilized through the formation of a number of lysine-derived intra- and intermolecular cross-links.

In some collagens (e.g., Type II), the three molecules are identical (the product of a single gene). In other collagens (e.g., Type I), two polypeptides of one kind (gene product) assemble with a second, quite similar, polypeptide, that is the product of a second gene. When the triple helix is secreted from the cell (usually by a fibroblast), the globular ends are cleaved off. The resulting linear, insoluble molecules assemble into collagen fibers. They assemble in a staggered pattern that gives rise to the striations (Figure 7).

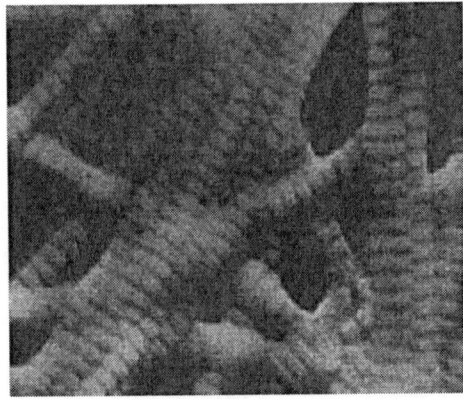

Figure 7. Staggered appearance of collagen.

Secondary and Tertiary Structure

The resulting molecule twists into an elongated, left-handed helix. When synthesized, the *N- terminal* and C- terminal of the polypeptide have globular domains, which keep the molecule soluble. As they pass through the endoplasmic reticulum (ER) and *Golgi apparatus,*

- The molecules are glycosylated.
- Hydroxyl (OH) groups are added to the "Y" amino acid.
- S-S bonds link three chains covalently.
- The three molecules twist together to form a triple helix.

The –OH group of hydroxy proline precipitates in inter chain hydrogen bonding through water molecule which in effect form a bridge between the chains. The hydrogen bonds contributed by hydroxy proline plays an important role in the stability of collagen since the triple helix is destroyed at temperature below the physiological temperature of 37°C, if the synthesis of hydroxy proline is inhibited. Other important factors in stabilizing the triple helix include electrostatic or ionic interactions between oppositely charged residues or adjacent chains, Vanderwall attraction, hydrophobic interaction, and covalent cross linking.

Biosynthesis of Collagen

Mesenchymal cells and their derivatives (fibroblasts, osteoblast, odontoblast, chondroblasts and cementoblasts) are the chief producers of collagen. Other cell types synthesizing collagen are epithelial, endothelial, muscle and Schwann cells.

Fibroblast

Fibroblast is the most common cell of connective tissue that produces and maintains the extracellular matrix. Fibroblasts provide a structural framework for many tissues and play an imperative role in wound healing. The key function of fibroblasts is to maintain the structural integrity of connective tissues by continuously secreting precursors of the extracellular matrix, primarily the ground substance and a variety of fibers. They are recognized by their association with collagen fibers bundles. The quiescent fibroblast or fibrocyte is smaller than the active fibroblast and is usually spindleshaped. It has fewer processes; a smaller, darker, elongated nucleus; and more acidophilic cytoplasm with much less rough endoplasmic reticulum. They have a branched cytoplasm surrounding an elliptical, speckled nucleus having one or two nucleoli. Active fibroblasts can be recognized by their oval, pale- staining nucleus and greater amount of cytoplasm, abundant rough endoplasmic reticulum, golgi apparatus, secretory vesicles and mitochondria. Fibroblasts exhibit contractility and motility which are important during connective tissue remodeling and formation and during wound repair. In certain tissues, fibroblasts have significant contractile properties and are called as myofibroblasts (Raines 2009)(Figure 8).

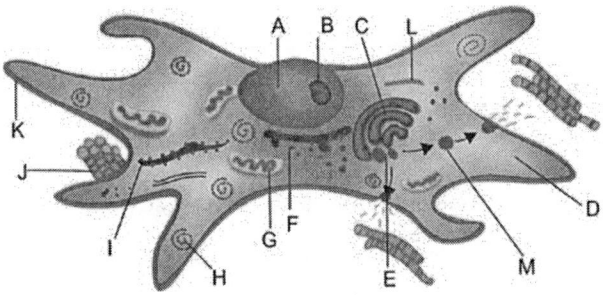

Figure 8. Structure of fibroblast. A: Nucleus; B: Nucleolus; C: Golgi apparatus; D: Cytoplasm; E; Intermediate/transfer vesicles; F: Ribosomes; G: Mitochondria; H: Polyribosomes; I: Rough Endoplasmic reticulum; J: Collagen fibrils; K: Cell processes; L: Microtubules; M: Secretory granules.

Biosynthesis of Collagen (Sandhu, Gupta, Singla 2012)

The individual collagen polypeptide chains are synthesized on the ribosome of the rough endoplasmic reticulum and secreted into the lumen, where they undergo complex enzymatic modifications prior to chain association and triple helix formation. The newly formed procollagen molecules are then secreted via secretory vacuoles originating from the golgi apparatus, and once in the extracellular space undergo further modification by specific proteinases which cleave off the N- and C-propeptides. The tropocollagen molecules thus formed may participate in fibril formation by aligning in a characteristic staggered array that is subsequently stabilized by the formation of covalent cross-links. –OH represents prolyl and lysyl hydroxylation.

The individual collagen polypeptide chains synthesize on the ribosome of the rough endoplasmic reticulum and are secreted into the lumen where they undergo complex enzymatic modifications prior to chain association and triple helix formation. The newly formed procollagen molecules then secrete via secretory vacuoles originating from the golgi apparatus, and once in the extracellular space undergo further modification by specific proteinases which cleave off the N- and C- pro peptides.

| Preprocollagen alpha chains are synthesized on RER (poses additional amino acid sequence called as propeptides at both amino acids and carboxyl ends are present). |

↓

| Preprocollagen enters cisternae of RER modified 1st signal sequence directing molecule to RER is removed followed by hydroxylation and glycosylation by addition of glucose and galactose |

↓

| Procollagen molecules are formed by alignment of three preprocollagen molecule with each other to form a light helical configuration. |

↓

| Procollagen molecules enter golgi apparatus via transfer vesiclesand modified further by addition of oligosaccharides. Modified procollagen molecule are packaged in trans golgi network and are immediately ferried out of cells. |

↓

| Formation and maintenance of fibrillary structures are augmented by covalent bonds formed between lysine and hydroxylysine residues of neighbouring tropocollagen molecules leading to formation collagen fibers which is catalysed by lysyl oxidase. |

↓

| As procollagen enters extracellular environment proteolytic enzyme procollagen peptidase, cleaves propeptides from amino and carboxyl ends. Newly formed molecule is shorter (280nm) in length called and is called as tropocollagen. |

Collagen gene

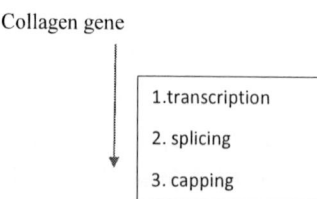

Figure 9. (Continued).

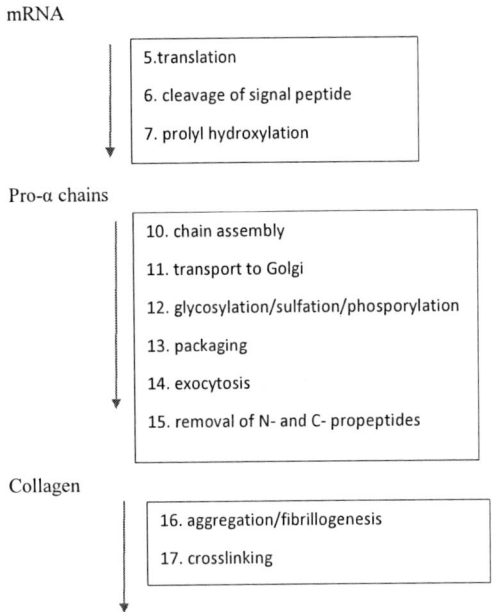

Figure 9. Steps in collagen formation.

The tropocollagen molecules thus formed may take part in fibril formation by aligning in a characteristic staggered array that subsequently stabilizes by the formation of covalent cross-links–OH represents prolyl and lysyl hydroxylation. Synthesis of collagen is a major aspect of developing tissues and it intimately involves in tissue differentiation, growth and remodeling. Young tissue exhibits high rates of collagen synthesis. As tissue matures in adults, synthesis continues as a part of normal tissue turnover. We observe the highest rates of collagen turnover in weight-bearing bones, periodontal ligament, lungs. Hormonal influences in reproductive tissues regulate the rate of collagen synthesis. Collagen synthesis elevates under conditions requiring remodeling and replacement of tissues. For instance, during tissue repair, such as wound and fracture healing, collagen synthesizes at elevated rates in pathological conditions such as fibrosis in lungs and liver. (Figure 9-11)

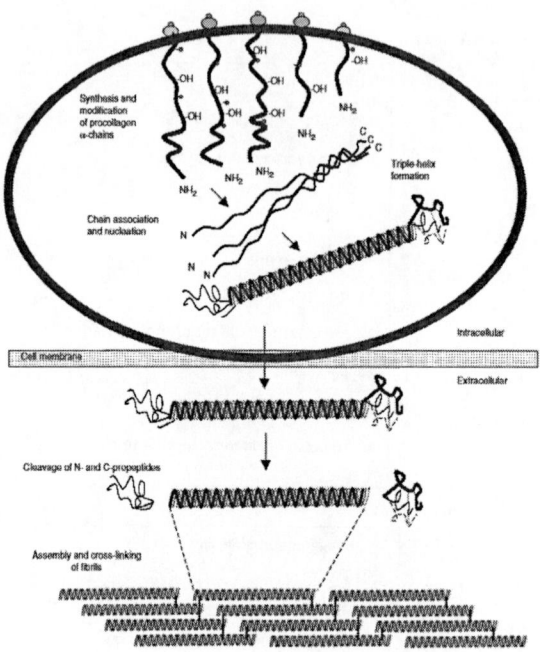

Figure 10. Schematic representation of the intercellular and extracellular steps involved in the synthesis, processing and assembly of type I collagen molecules into fibrils.

Cells which Synthesize Collagen

Collagen is synthesized by cells of mesodermal origin collectively referred as fibroblasts. In highly differentiated state, these cells acquire characteristics especially suited to the chemistry of the tissue. Examples are chondroblasts in cartilage, odontoblasts in the teeth and osteoblast in bones. Collagen synthesizing cells are characterized by an extensive rough endoplasmic reticulum (RER) and well developed Golgi apparatus like other proteins. Collagen is synthesized on the RER and the completed molecules are related into cisternae from which they pass into the golgi apparatus and secreted into the cellular space because of its usual physico-chemical properties and chemical composition the synthesis of collagen involves many steps not observed in the biosynthesis of other proteins.

1. Collagen is not soluble under physiological conditions.
2. Aggregation of collagen molecules occurs very soon after the molecules are synthesized.
3. Collagen must be kept in a soluble state until it is reaches fibrillogenesis.
4. Another important consideration is the presence of hydroxyproline, hydrolysine, and hydrolysine glycosides.

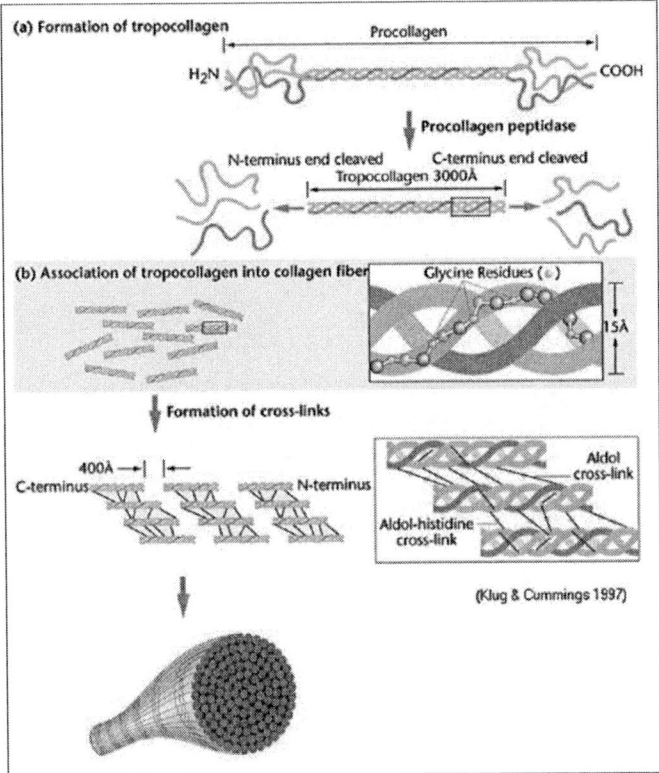

Figure 11. Formation of collagen

The two amino acids, hydroxy proline and hydroxylysine in a post translation phase are modified from peptides proline and lysine. This modification occurs only on nacent α chains because the triple helical collagen molecule is not accessible to the modification enzymes. Some collagen molecules contain sugar residue at the triple helical domain and other have covalently attached glycosaminoglycan chains. For these reasons, the collagen molecule is first synthesized as a larger precursor containing extra amino acids at both N and C terminal ends. Synthesis of these pro α-chains, their assembly into procollagen and their conversion into collagen fibers involves several well-coordinated biosynthetic reactions occurring in the nucleus, cytoplasm, and extracellular space.

Types of Collagen: (Bartold PM 1988)

The collagen family is composed of 28 collagen types and 38 genetically distinct α-chains, four of which are under characterization. (Table 1, Figure 10, 11)

They are mainly divided into 3 groups:

Group I

These are fibrillar collagen or fibril forming collagen. It includes Type I, II, III, V and XI. The most easily recognized forms of collagens are those that form banded fibrils, and we call these fibrils-forming collagens. Type I, II, III, V, and- XI collagens belong to this group. In these molecules, the triple helical domain contains an uninterrupted stretch of 338 to 343. Gly-X-Y triplets in each α chain, and the molecule measures 15 x 3000

Group II

These are fibril associated collagens with interrupted triple helix (FACIT). These groups of collagen comprise proteins in which non-collagenous sequence interrupt the collagen. They are associated with the surface fibril-forming collagens. It includes Type IX, XII, XIV, XVI.

Group III

All other non-fibrillar collagen form the third group which include:

1) Network forming collagen: Type IV, VIII, X.
2) Beaded collagen - type VI
3) Anchoring fibrils Type VII (Figure 12)

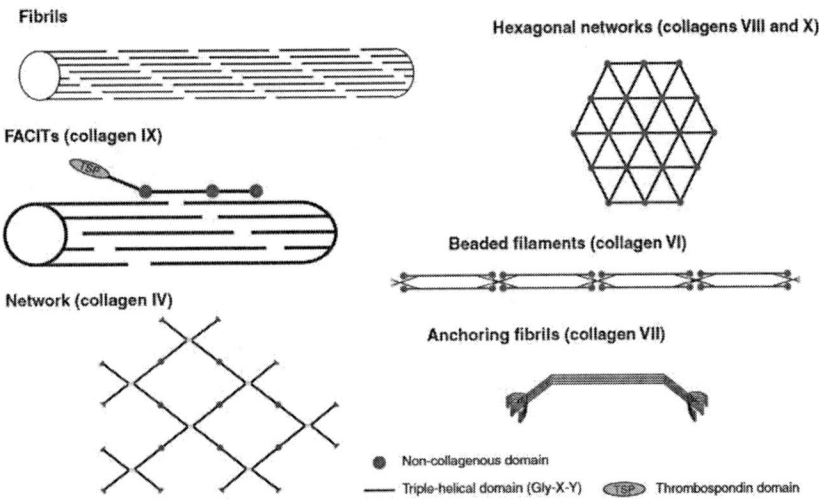

Figure 12. Various types of collagen fibrils.

These collagen forms sheets or protein membranes enclosing tissues and organs. In addition to the above collagen groups, at least ten noncollagenous proteins incorporating short, triple helical collagen domains have been described. This group of collagen domain-containing non-matrix proteins includes the C1q component of C1 complement, lung surfactant protein, acetylcholinesterase, conglutinin, and mannose binding protein. These proteins are not considered true collagen because they do not form a part of the extracellular matrix.

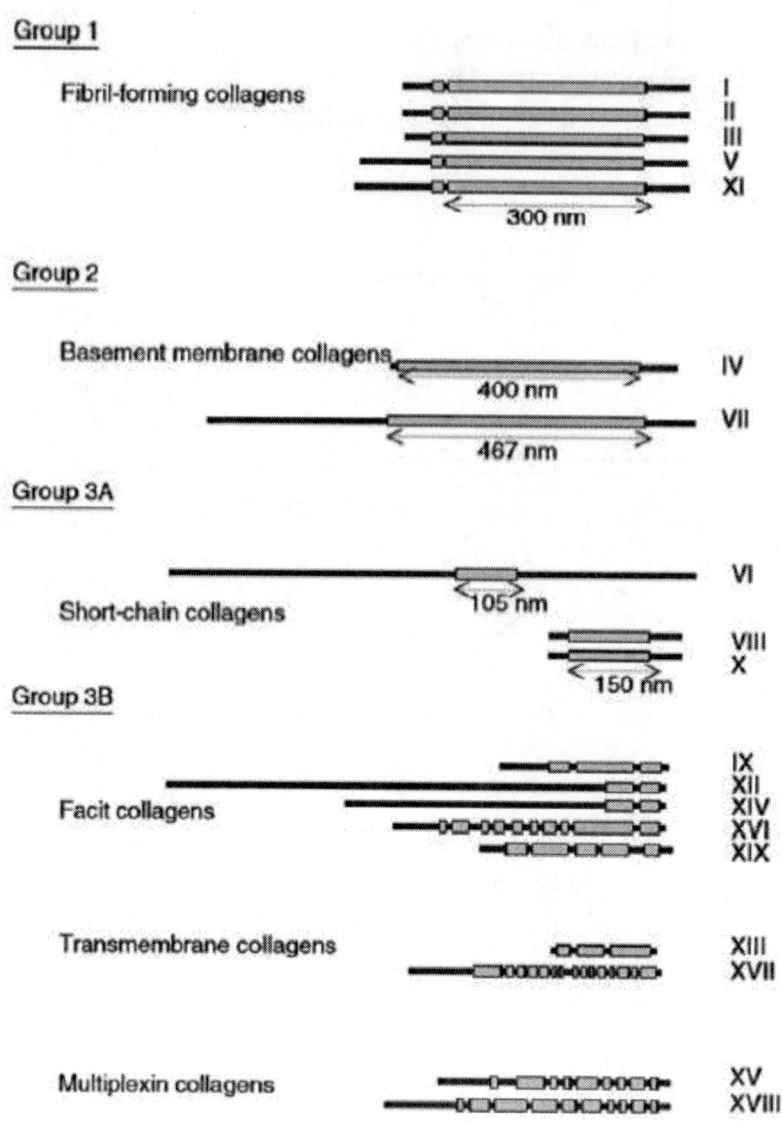

Figure 13. Group of collagen fibrils

Table 1. Types of Collagen

Type	Constituent	Chain composition	Occurrence
I	α1(I)	[α1(I)]$_2$α2(I) common	Most connective tissues; abundant in dermis, bone, tendon, ligament, cornea
	α2(I)	[α1(I)]$_3$ rare	
II	α1(II)	[α1(II)]$_3$	Cartilage, vitreous body
III	α1(III)	[α1(III)]$_3$	Tissues rich in collagen I, especially skin, blood vessels, and inner organs; not in bone or cartilage
IV	α1(IV)	[α1(IV)]$_2$α2(IV)	All basement membranes
	α2(IV)	[α3(IV)]$_3$	
	α3(IV)	[α3(IV)]$_2$α4(IV)	
	α4(IV)	α3(IV)α4(IV)α5(IV)	
	α5(IV)	α1(IV)?α6(IV)?	
	α6(IV)	α3(IV)?α6(IV)?	
V	α1(V)	[α1(V)]$_2$α2(V)	Tissues containing collagen I; quantitatively minor component
	α2(V)	α1(V)α2(V)α3(V)	
	α3(V)	[α1(V)]$_3$	
	α4(V)	α1(V)?α4(V)?	
VI	α1(VI)	α1(VI)α2(VI)α3(VI)	Most connective tissues, including cartilage
	α2(VI)		
	α3(VI)		
VII	α1(VII)	[α1(VII)]$_3$	Anchoring fibrils (skin, cornea, cervix, oral and oesophageal mucosa)
VIII	α1(VIII)	[α1(VIII)]$_2$α2(VIII)	Many tissues, e.g., Descemet's membrane of eye (Greenhill et al., 2000)
	α2(VIII)	[α1(VIII)]$_3$, [α2(VIII)]$_3$	
IX	α1(IX)	α1(IX)α2(IX)α3(IX)	Tissues containing type II collagen; quantitatively minor component
	α2(IX)		
	α3(IX)		
X	α1(X)	[α1(X)]$_3$	Hypertrophic cartilage
XI	α1(XI)	α1(XI)α2(XI)α3(XI)	Tissues containing collagen II; quantitatively minor component
	α2(XI)	other forms	
	α3(XI)§		
XII	α1(XII)	[α1(XII)]$_3$	Tissues containing collagen I; quantitatively minor component
XIII	α1(XIII)	[α1(XIII)]$_3$	Most tissues in low quantities
XIV	α1(XIV)	[α1(XIV)]$_3$	Tissues containing collagen I; quantitatively minor component
XV	α1(XV)	ND	Many tissues in the BM zone
XVI	α1(XVI)	[α1(XVI)]$_3$	Many tissues
XVII	α1(XVII)	[α1(XVII)]$_3$	Skin hemidesmosomes
XVIII	α1(XVIII)	ND	Many tissues in the BM zone
XIX	α1(XIX)	ND	Many tissues in the BM zone

Table 1. (Continued)

Type	Constituent	Chain composition	Occurrence
* Fibril-forming collagen-like			
* FACIT-like, XXI (Fitzgerald & Bateman, 2001)			mRNAs in many tissues, incl. heart, stomach, kidney, skeletal muscle, placenta
* FACIT-like			
* Collagen XIII-like			

Arrangement of Collagen Fibres in Various Tissues (Gelse, Pöschl, and Aigner 2003)

All tissues contain a mixture of several collagen types. Type I is the most abundant collagen in mammalian tissue. It accounts for 65% to 95% of the total collagens. Type III is the second major species in soft connective tissue and its proportion ranges from 5% to 30% in adult tissue and higher in fetal and granulation tissue. These two types of collagen are co-distributed with the minor collagen like Type V, VI, XII, and XIV. The major function of type I and III collagen is to provide mechanical strength to the tissues. Among the calcified tissue, bone contains predominantly Type I collagen together with very small quantities of Type V, III, XII, and XIV. In cartilage, type II is the major fibril forming collagen with other minor species including type XI and FACIT types IX, XII. Type II collagen is necessary for mechanical strength in cartilage. Type IX collagen permits cartilage to function at low friction by coating the articular surface. Type IV collagen is found only in basement membrane structure. This collagen is bound to anchoring fibrils of type VII collagen. (Figure 12,13)

Distinctive Features of Various Types of Collagen (Table 1)

- **Type I collagen:** It forms fibrillar arrangement with fibres of high tensile strength. This type of collagen has relatively little carbohydrate associated with α-chains, and less than 10% hydroxyl lysine per chain. Broad fibrils have a single molecule (J) with a mol. wt. of 285kd.
- **Type II Collagen:** It forms fibrous aggregates which are spares in comparison to type I collagen. It has large amount of carbohydrate. It has more than 20% of hydroxylysine per chain. Fibrils are usually thinner than type I.
- **Type III Collagen:** It forms fibrils but less than type I. Type III collagen has been found only in association with Type I collagen and in tissue which support an endothelium or epithelium. It has significant amount of cystine, low carbohydrate, high hydroxy proline and glycine.
- **Type IV collagen:** It is the collagen of basement membrane, containing greater amount of hydroxy proline and hydroxy lysine, 40% per chain and cystine than any other collagen. It contain 3 hydroxy proline in addition to 4-hydroxy proline which appears in all collagen.

Structural formula is:

$$\begin{array}{c} \text{COOH} \\ | \\ \text{CH-NH}_2 \ (\alpha\text{-Amino acids}) \\ | \\ \text{R} \end{array}$$

Commonly occurring amino acids are twenty in number. Most of the amino acids except proline are α–amino acids, which mean that the amino group is attached to the same carbon atom to which carboxyl group is attached.

Glycine: Simplest amino acids, non-essential, hydrophilic, Glucogenic, mol. Wt. 77D, average occurrence in protein is 7.5%.

Cysteine: Sulphur containing amino acids, non-essential, hydrophobic, glucogenic, mol. Wt. 121 D, average occurrence in protein is 2.8%. It contains pyrrolidine group, since it has a secondary amino group it is called as imino acid, non-essential, hydrophobic, lipophilic, glucogenic, mol. Wt. 115D, average occurrence in protein 4.6%.

Lysine: Is diabasic mono carboxylic acid, essential amino acid, partially ketogenic and partially glucogenic, mol. Wt. 146D, average occurrence in protein is 7%.

Hydroxy proline and Hydroxy Lysine: These are important component of collagen, which are derived amino acids found in protein. The main role of amino acid is in the synthesis of structural and functional proteins.

Peptide Bond

Alpha carboxyl group of one amino acid reacts with α amino group of another amino acid to form a peptide bond or CO-NH bridge. Proteins are made by polymerization of amino acids through peptide bonds. Two amino acids are combined to form dipeptide. Few amino acids together will make an oligopeptide. Combination of 10-50 amino acids is called as polypeptide and polypeptide chain containing more than 50 amino acids are called proteins.

In a tripeptide, there are three amino acids but these three can be any of the total 20 amino acids so 8000 different permutation and combinations are possible in a tripeptide. An ordinary protein having about 100 amino acids will have 20 or 100 different possibilities. This is more than the no. of stars in the milkyway galaxy. Thus even though there are only 20 amino acids, by changing the sequence of combination of these amino acids nature produce enormous number of different proteins. Peptide bond is a partials double bond. It is a rigid and planar and there is no freedom of rotation. The angle of rotation is known as Ramachandran Angle.

End Groups of Polypeptide Chains

In a polypeptide chain at one end there will be one free α-amino group, this end is called amino terminal or N-terminal and the amino acids contributing the α-amino group is named as the first amino acid. The other end of polypeptide chain is the carboxy terminal end, C-terminal. All other α-amino and carboxyl groups are involved in peptide bond formation. Usually N-terminal amino acid is written on the left hand side when the sequence of protein is denoted incidentally the biosynthesis of protein also starts from the amino terminal end.

Amino Acid Composition of Collagen

Each polypeptide chain of collagen has about 1050 amino acid residues. The amino acid composition of collagen is quite unique. About 1/3 rd of the amino acid is glycine that is every third residue is glycine. Glycine forms 33% of total protein. Others are proline which is 10% and other derived amino acids like hydroxy proline, 10% and hydroxy lysine, 1%. Predominant forms of hydroxyl proline is 4-OH derivatives although some type of collagen contains small amount of 3-OH proline.

Small amount of carbohydrate is found in collagen covalently bound through carbohydrate (0.4-12% by wt) located in hole region. Gly makes strong H2 bond with carboxyl O_2 of an X residue of neighboring chain.

Amino Acid Sequence of Collagen

The molecular unit of collagen in collagen fibrils is the tropocollagen molecule. Each tropocollagen molecule contains three polypeptide chains. In the tropocollagen of some three types each of the three polypeptide chain has an identical amino acid sequence.

Ex: In Type II collagen: (α1 (II))3
Type III collagen: (α1 (III))3
Type IV collagen: (α1 (IV))3

In Type I collagen, two of the chains are identical in sequence and the amino acid sequence of third chain differ slightly. The amino acid sequence of the polypeptide strands in the tropocollagen molecule is also quite different. The repetitive amino acid sequence may be represented by (Gly-x-y-Gly-x-y), X and Y are other amino acids most commonly proline, hydroxy proline. Except for a small segment of 15 to 25 amino acids, on the NH2 and COOH terminal ends. These segments are known as Telopeptides. Glycine is found in every third amino acid in the sequence. Further more the sequence Gly-Pro-Y and Gly-H-Xyp, X and y are any of the amino acids 5 .Glycine pass through center of the triple helix. Only Gly fit at the center. Each repeated about 100 times in the polypeptide sequence of chain. These two triples sequence will encompass about 600 amino acids within a tropocollagen chain of approximately 1000 amino acids. Approximately 100 of X residues are proline and 100 of Y residues are 4-hydroxy proline.

CHARACTERISTIC FEATURES OF COLLAGEN

1) The presence of triple helical structure formed by three polypeptide chains called α - chains are left handed helix of 3 residues per turn which wrap around each other into a right handed rope like triple helical rod of 15A° diameter and 3000A° long. Depending upon the type of collagen, the molecule may be made up of either three identical α -chains or two identical chains or three different α -chains. The triple helix may be a continuous stretch or it may be interrupted by non –collagenous segments.
2) The alternate dark and light bonds that appear 670A° along the long axis of the super coiled tropocollagen molecule is called as D periodicity.
3) Within the triple helix glycine occupies every third portion in the repeating amino acid sequence Gly-x-y, where x and y are usually amino acids other than glycine. Glycine is essential for triple helical conformation because larger amino acids will not fit in the

center of the triple helix. Proline, hydroxy proline frequently occupies the x and y position.

4) Collagen contains two unique amino acids proline, hydroxy proline and hydroxy lysine. These amino acids are present in y position.
5) Collagen molecule is stabilized by the formation of a number of lysine derived intra and inter molecular cross link.
6) Collagen contains more glycine than any other vertebrate protein.
7) Glycine residue occurs at the crossing point.
8) Proline and hydroxy proline accounts for nearly $(1/4)^{th}$ of the total residue.
9) Collagen contains cytine only in type III and IV collagen chains. In addition to amino acids collagen also contains carbohydrates. Carbohydrates are galactose and glycose bound to hydroxy lysine group. Amount of carbohydrate varies from tissue to tissue and differ in chain types. They help in Fibrillogenesis. They may regulate interactions between collagen molecules and between collagen and other structural macro molecules.

Morphological Characteristics

In the body, Type I, II and III collagen always occur in the form of fibres of varying dimensions. Type I forming largest fibres, appear to the naked eye as glistening pearly white strands. In electron microscopy they appear as beaded thread like structure. When it is stained with appropriate electron dense material, the fibre exhibits a highly regular, transversely bonded pattern with a periodicity or repeat distance D of 68nm of 680A°. This axial repeat is nearly constant in all organisms. Collagen fibres are essentially cylindrical in cross-section diameter (4A° to 4000A°). The fibres in various tissues are present in bundles or interwoven in different pattern according to the properties and functions. They have the rigidity and ability to bear high impact and mechanical stress in bone.

Diameter of collagen fibre is 100A°-2000A°. That arises from the presence of collagen in complex with proteoglycans and hydroxy apatite crystals. The fibres are highly ordered aggregates of the individual molecules of collagens which are rigid rod like structures, each approximately 300nm or 3000A° long and 1.5 nm or 15A° diameter. 68nm or 680A° axial repeat (D) is generated by the staggering of the molecules along their long axis. The length of the molecule is 4.4D. A two dimensional arrangement in which adjacent molecules are staggered by the repeat distance (D) was suggested by Petruska and Hodge.

This type of arrangement lead to a structure with gaps of some 30 nm between ends of the molecule and an overlap region. This explains the light and dark band seen in low power electron microscope.

Gene Expression (Vuorio 1990)

Collagen genes are large and range in size from 5kb for COL 1AL to 130kb for Col 13Al. They are several times as large as their respectives mRnas. More than 30 genes have been described for collagen type I to XIX. Those for fibril forming collagen have a similar exon arrangement and these genes contain H2 exons for the major triple helical region. Most of these exons are composed of 54bp and start with an intact coden for glycine. However the organization of non fibrillar collagen gene vary for example exams for the type IV collagen genes do not confirm to the 54bp rule and they frequently start with a split coden for glycine in this collagen the COL4A5-Col4A6 the Col4A3 – Col4A4 and the Col4A5-Col4A6 genes are arranged in a unique head to head orientation separated by nucleotides. Sequences in the size of exons in type IX collagen ranges from 21 to 400bp. Type VI collagen gene is composed of only 34 exons.

Structurally, the collagen genes, like other genes, can be roughly divided into two categories based on the characteristics in their core promoter areas. These categories are "tissue-specific genes," which have TATA boxes specifying the precise position of transcription initiation, and "housekeeping genes," which lack TATA boxes, but have instead high GC-contents and multiple transcription start sites.

The genes belonging into the latter category are transcribed widely in many tissues, but at low RNA levels. Of the collagen genes, those encoding the major fibrillar collagens, COL1A1, COL2A1, and COL3A1, the COL10A1 encoding the highly specialized collagen of hypertrophic chondrocytes, and the downstream promoter initiating the synthesis of the cornea-specific transcript of collagen IX belong to the tissue-specific gene category. COL4A3-A4, COL5A1, COL7A1, COL9A2-A3, COL11A1, COL11A2, Col13a, the promoter 1 of Col18a, and the downstream promoter of COL6A2 all belong to the housekeeping genes category.

Furthermore, some collagen promoters, such as COL4A5-6 and the promoter 2 of Col18a, lack both TATA- and GC-boxes, but contain CCAAT boxes. Others, however, lack all the above mentioned proximal promoter elements, and examples of these are COL6A1 and the upstream promoter of the cartilage-specific transcript of collagen IX.

Translation and Posttranslational Events

Collagen mRNAs are transcribed as precursors and undergo the usual processing reactions, including capping, polyadenylation, and splicing. After these nuclear events, the mRNA is translocated to the cytoplasm where it binds to ribosomes and gets translated. The mRNA codes for the pre-pro-a chain, which (in type I, II, and III collagens) contains approximately 1500 amino acids, and includes the signal sequence and extra N- and C-terminal sequences not present in mature α chains. Signal sequences are cleaved during polypeptide chain elongation as the nascent pro-a chains are being transported into the rough endoplasmic reticulum (RER) lumen. As translation of the pro-a (pre-pro-a minus the signal peptide) proceeds, cenain prolyl and lysyl residues at the Y position are oxidized to Hyp and Hyl, respectively, by enzymes. Prolyl hydroxylation is performed, predominantly at the C-4 position, by the enzyme prolyl-4hydroxylase. This enzyme is a tetramer consisting of two a and two subunits, with molecular masses of 64 and 60 kd, respectively. Some prolyl residues are hydroxylated at C-3 to 3-Hyp by a different enzyme, prolyl3-hydroxylase. The lysyl hydroxylase is a homodimer of 85-kd subunits. These hydroxylases require Zn + Fe ++, α -ketoglutarate, and ascorbic acid (vitamin C) as cofactors. Only nascent pro-a chains act as substrates for these enzymes, not triple helical molecules.

The minimum amino acid sequence requirement for prolyl hydroxylation is X-Pro-Gly. All available prolyl and lysyl residues are not hydroxylated; the extent of hydroxylation depends upon the availability of substrate, type of tissue, and other factors. The relative rate and extent of hydroxylation also vary between collagen types. For example, in type IV collagen, 3-prolyl hydroxylation occurs to a higher degree than in types I, II, and III, with up to 90% of its lysines hydroxylated.

Triple helical type I collagen, with fully hydroxylated 4-hydroxyproline, has a Tm (melting temperature, above which the collagen triple helix is denatured to a chains) of 39°C. However, underhydroxylated molecules melt at lower temperatures, and the Tm of completely unhydroxylated collagen is 25°C. Therefore, prolyl hydroxylation is essential for collagen thermal stability at physiologic temperature, while underhydroxylated molecules are denatured and degraded.

Hydroxylysine residues, on the other hand, serve as specific glycyosylation sites, and form more stable cross-links than lysine. The role of 3-hydroxyproline, however, is unclear.

The pro- α chains undergo glycosylation at certain Hyl and Asn residues during translation, and oligosaccharides rich in galactose, galactose plus glucose (to hydroxylysine), or mannose (to asparagine) are added. Glycosylation occurs at the C-5 oxygen of peptidyl hydroxylysine and it is carried out by the enzymes hydroxylysylgalactosyl transferase and galactosyl hydroxylysy lglucosyl transferase. These enzymes transfer UDP-galactose and UDP-glucose, respectively. The glycosylation of hydroxylysyl residues takes place in the RER lumen, and oligosaccharides are added to asparagine residues in the ER and Golgi complex.

As soon as the synthesis of pro-a chains is completed, two pro α 1 (I) chains and one pro α 2(I) in type I, or three pro α chains in collagen types

II and III, associate at the C-terminal ends. This association is stabilized by interchain disulfide bond formation, which is catalyzed by the enzyme protein-disulfide isomerase. Triple helix formation is thus initiated and proceeds from the C-terminal toward the N-terminal end, like a zipper. The rate of collagen folding is limited by the extent of cistrans isomerization of prolyl bonds. Collagen chain assembly and folding of types I and IV collagens involve the heat shock protein Hsp47 as a molecular chaperone. Some procollagens lack large C-terminal domains (e.g., type XII), and these pro collagens appear to fold by mechanisms not involving the formation of a nucleus at the C-terminus.

The pro collagen molecule thus assembled is then translocated to the Golgi complex, where additional glycosylation and phosphorylation may occur. Sulfate (e.g., in type V) and phosphate (to type I in bone) groups may also be added to tyrosyl and seryl residues, respectively, located at the N-terminal pro peptide domain. The pro collagen molecules are then packaged into vesicles, which fuse with cell membrane and release their contents into the extracellular space.

DISEASES ASSOCIATED WITH COLLAGEN ALTERATIONS

Since most tissues contain a blend of collagen types, any adjustment in the structure, substance, or extent of collagen types can be relied upon to prompt utilitarian variations from the norm of the tissues containing these collagens. Three sorts of modifications can influence collagens and lead to connective tissue changes: an imperfection in the structure of collagen qualities, a sub-atomic deformity in the preparing catalysts, and systems influencing the statement of collagen qualities because of pathologies of acquired diseases.

Diseases because of molecular defects are inherited, and those related with acquired diseases, despite the fact that they may include at least one hereditary component are induced by a variety of physiologic and environmental factors.

Inherited Diseases of Collagen Structure and Biosynthesis

These diseases emerge because of point mutations, deletions, or insertions in the structural genes for collagens or their posttranslational processing enzymes. The severity of these diseases relies upon a few elements. For type I collagen, mutations that affect the assembly of pro α 1 (I) chains can be lethal, whereas those affecting pro α 2(I) assembly are not lethal.

This distinction emerges in light of the fact that homodimers of α 1 (I) formed in the absence of pro α 2(I) are stable at physiologic temperature, whereas the α 2(I)3 formed in the absence of α 1 (I) isn't steady and gets degraded. In this manner, large deletions, insertions, or mutations near the C-terminus of pro- α 1 (I), which influence its assembly into collagen, are often lethal. Replacement of glycine with other amino acids diminishes the rate of collagen folding, its thermal stability, and secretion; therefore, such mutant molecules are held intracellularly for a more extended period and are degraded. Mutations associated with the genes of collagen-processing enzymes, however, are usually not lethal, despite the fact that they lead to functional abnormalities of constituent tissues.

Very nearly 200 transformations have been described in COL1A1 and COL1A2 genes up until now, and many of these mutations have been associated with various forms of osteogenesis imperfecta and Ehlers-Danlos syndrome (EDS).

Osteogenesis Imperfecta (Kierszenbaum AL 2002, Gupte et al. 2017)

Osteogenesis imperfecta is a heterogeneous group of disorders associated with bone fragility, dentinogenesis imperfecta, hearing loss, blue sclera, and soft tissue dysplasia. It is subdivided into four major subclasses.

Osteogenesis imperfecta type 1 is a dominantly inherited form with blue sclera, but normal teeth and near-normal stature. It is caused most commonly by mutations that decrease type 1 procollagen production because of mutations that lead to null COL1A1 alleles. Other molecular defects identified in this disease incorporate substitution of glycine by cysteine, particularly close to the N-terminal end.

Osteogenesis imperfecta type II is lethal in the perinatal period, and this disease is associated with new dominant mutations. This form arises due to mutations that affect pro collagen assembly by substitution of glycine near the C-terminal end, rearrangement of multiple exons bringing about loss of an enormous portion of amino acids, or mutations at the C-terminal propeptide of pro α (I). Osteogenesis imperfecta type III is a genetically heterogeneous disease most commonly inherited in autosomal dominant, and once in a while as recessive, forms, and it is a progressively deforming variety.

Point mutations in pro α 1 (I) genes, and mutations in pro α 2(1) that prevent its inclusion in collagen molecules, have been identified as some of the causes for this disease. Osteogenesis imperfecta type N is a dominantly inherited disease caused by point mutations and small deletions in the α 2(1) gene; a typical component of this sort of osteogenesis imperfecta is dentinogenesis imperfecta.

Ehlers-Danlos Syndrome (Yen et al. 2006, Letourneau Y, Perusse R 2001)

The Ehlers-Danlos syndrome represents another heterogeneous group of connective tissue diseases characterized by skin fragility and hyper extensibility, and hypermobility of the joints. Among these, the Ehlers-Danlos syndrome type IV i.e., the vascular, or ecchymotic, type, is characterized by arterial rupture and spontaneous rupture of the colon, and the defects identified in this disease are mutations or multiple exon deletions within the COL3A1 gene.

In Ehlers-Danlos syndrome type VI, ocular form in which blindness and kyphoscoliosis are significant highlights, lysyl hydroxylase activity is severely depressed, and lysines in type I and III collagens, but not in type

II and IV, are underhydroxylated. In Ehlers-Danlos syndrome type VII, the defect is impairment of the procollagen-to-collagen conversion. In this disease, the assembly of collagens into functional fibrils is influenced due to steric hindrance by the retained pro-peptide domain. The transformation may be impaired due to mutations at the N-propeptidase cleavage site exon 6 of COL1A1 or COL1A2.

This is the defect in Ehlers-Danlos syndrome forms VIIA and B. On the other hand, the enzyme itself may be affected; this is the defect in Ehlers-Danlos syndrome form VIIC (dermatosparaxis). EhlersDanlos syndrome type VIII is an autosomal dominant form described by periodontal involvement and loss of teeth; the molecular defect responsible for this disease has not yet been identified. Marked reduction in the activity of lysyl oxidase, due to defective intracellular distribution of copper, a cofactor for lysyl oxidase, gives rise to Ehlers-Danlos syndrome type IX (cutis laxa or occipital horn syndrome). This is an X-linked recessive disease.

In the type II collagen gene (COL2A1), around 50 mutations that lead to chondrodysplasias have been accounted for. The chondrodysplasias are a heterogeneous group of diseases portrayed by abnormal growth or development of cartilage, and their severity ranges from mild symptoms to perinatal death.

Three significant types of this group of disorders are achondrogenesis/hypochondrogenesis, spondyloepiphyseal dysplasia, and Stickler syndrome. Individuals affected by these diseases show abnormalities in type II collagen-containing tissues such as growth plates, and vitreous humor.

The type of mutations identified in these diseases are similar to those for type I collagen, and include a glycine-to-aspartate substitution in a Kniest dysplasia, an arginineto-cysteine conversion, and a fascinating Gto-T transversion that interferes with splicing and results in the deletion of 18 amino acids. Mutations in type X collagen, a product of hypertrophic chondrocyres, cause a type of dwarfism known as Schmid metaphyseal chondrodysplasia in humans. Molecular defects have also been described in the basement membrane collagens. Alport syndrome is a progressive hereditary nephritis related with senso-neuronal deafness and ocular abnormalities. It has an X-linked inheritance pattern, and it is characterized by splitting and thinning of the glomerular basement membrane. This condition has been connected to defects on the COL4A5 gene. Point mutations in triple helical and C-propeptide domains and multiple exon deletions have been recognized as the etiological factors. Mutations have additionally been distinguished in COL7 Al gene in individuals affected by the dominantly or recessively inherited forms of dystrophic epidermolysis bullosa. In this disease dermal-epidermal integrity is affected due to abnormal or absent anchoring fibrils, and the molecular defects are in the type VII collagen gene. The degree of association of periodontal structures in collagen molecular diseases ranges from slight to significant, exception for dentinogenesis imperfecta, molecular defects in other diseases have not been investigated in detail.

Stickler Syndrome (Rose et al. 2001)

It is an extraordinary autosomal dominant syndrome of premature osteoarthritis, retinal degeneration, hearing loss and orofacial abnormalities described by Gunnar B Stickler in 1965. The disorder (hereditary arthro-ophthalmopathy or Stickler syndrome) is known to be caused by mutations in the COL2A1, COL11A1 and COL11A2 procollagen genes of type 2 and 11 collagen.

Alport Syndrome (Kashtan 2017)

Alport syndrome is a generalized inherited disorder of basement membranes, particularly those of glomeruli that involve type IV collagen. The mutations occur in the gene located on the X chromosome. Inherited defect of the classical X-linked Alport syndrome affects the α-5 chain of collagen type IV collagen gene (COL4A5) while the α-3 and α-4 chain of collagen type IV collagen gene (COL4A3 and COL4A4) are liable for less frequent recessive forms of Alport syndrome. It is characterized by renal impairment, loss of hearing and lens abnormalities, hypertension, hematuria and proteinuria. The damage of collagen IV due to mutations causes dysfunction of bound epithelium and results in organ damage.

Epidermolysis Bullosa (Neville BW, Damm DD, Allen CM 2009) (Al-Jobeir 2006)

Hereditary epidermolysis bullosa is a group of rare genetically transmitted disorders that have several methods of inheritance with various degrees of severity and expression. It is a multiracial disorder that is characterized by the formation of vesicles and bullae on the skin and mucous membranes. The vesicles may emerge spontaneously or from minor trauma. The four types of epidermolysis bullosa are simplex, dystrophic and junctional and hemidesmosomal. Specific mutations in the K5 or K14 genes and genes coding for the laminin has been responsible for dominant simplex type and junctional form respectively. The dystrophic type is related with mutations in the type VII gene. The hemidesmosomal type is described by mutations of genes associated with various hemidesmosomal attachment proteins such as plectin, type XVII collagen and α6β4 integrin.

Marfan Syndrome (Al-Mulla 2013)

It is the most widely recognized inherited connective tissue disorder with a reported incidence of one in 10,000 individual and equivalent disseminations between the gendersIt is brought about by an autosomal dominant mutation in the gene encoding fibrillin (FBN1, chromosome 15q15–21.3), a glycoprotein that is a vital piece of the connective tissue in the body (ligaments, blood vessel, eye lenses). It fundamentally includes the skeletal, ocular and cardiovascular systems. Commonly, patients present with tall stature, ectopia lentis, aortic root dilatation and a positive family history. The diagnosis is made when a patient present with complications of the syndrome, such as aortic dissection or with involvement of the pulmonary, skin/integument or nervous systems.

Autoimmune Collagen Disorders

1. Systemic lupus erythematosus (Neville BW, Damm DD, Allen CM 2009) (Lourenço et al. 2007): Lupus erythematosus is a

multifactorial autoimmune collagen vascular or connective tissue disease, which may also impact the oral mucosa in both its cutaneous and systemic forms with varied prevalence. Common findings consist of fever, weight loss, arthritis, fatigue and general malaise. A characteristic rash, having the example of a butterfly, develops over the malar region and nose. Cardiac involvement is also common with pericarditis. Warty vegetations affecting the coronary heart valves (Libman-Sacks endocarditis) are also observed. Oral lesions consist of ulceration, pain, erythema and hyperkeratosis may be present. Other oral complaints are xerostomia, stomatodynia, candidiasis, periodontal disease and dysgeusia.

2. Systemic sclerosis (Neville BW, Damm DD, Allen CM 2009)(Cazal et al. 2008) (progressive systemic sclerosis; scleroderma; hide-bound disease): Progressive systemic sclerosis is a disorder of the connective tissue that illustrates fibrosis of the skin, blood vessels, visceral organs and mucosa. The precise mechanism of the fibrotic changes is unknown however hyperplastic changes of collagen have been documented. The pathological findings characterise that fibroblasts are activated to produce immoderate amounts of collagen and other components of the cellular matrix. The most apparent symptom is the involvement of the skin together with the quality of its mobility, particularly in the distal portions of the extremities. Cutaneous manifestations consist of thickening of skin, beginning with pitting edema and over several months pitting edema is replaced by tightening and hardening of skin. Raynaud's phenomenon is usually the first symptom. The oral manifestations consist of classic facial skin hardening and limited opening of the oral orifice with characteristic furrows radiating from the mouth resulting in a classic mask-like and purse string appearance respectively. Bone resorption at the angle of the mandible is also a common feature. Deposition of collagen within the lingual and esophageal

submucosa, producing a firm, hypomobile (board-like) tongue and an inelastic esophagus, thus resulting in dysphagia.
3. Oral submucous fibrosis: It is a chronic, premalignant condition of the oral mucosa which was first described by Schwartz 1952. Recently it is thought to be an autoimmune disease. The presence of diverse autoantibodies in varying titers is reported in several studies confirming autoimmune basis to the disease.(Gupta, Mhaske, and Ragavendra 2008) Tilakratne WM et al. in 2006 reported that even though the data on numerous HLA types, raised autoantibodies and the detection of immune complexes tend to signify an autoimmune foundation for the disease substantial range of cases and matched controls may be required to verify these findings (Tilakaratne et al. 2006). This disease is considered to be an effect of disturbances in the homeostatic equilibrium between synthesis and degradation of extracellular matrix, in which collagen forms a major component, as a result it can be identified as a collagen-metabolic disorder. It is characterized by a juxta epithelial inflammatory reaction followed by fibroelastic change in the lamina propria and associated epithelial atrophy. This leads to a restricted mouth opening, resulting in trismus leading to restriction of food consumption, difficulty in maintaining oral health, as well as impairs the ability to speak. The fibroelastic changes are almost entirely because of abnormal accumulation of collagen in the subepithelial layers, resulting in dense fibrous bands in the mouth (Shukla, Kumar, and Kumar 2017) (Rajalalitha and Vali 2005).

Scurvy

A deficiency of vitamin C is called as scurvy. The main function of ascorbic acid is its involvement in the synthesis of collagen fibers from proline via hydroxyproline. Other metabolic reactions for which vitamin C is needed are the hydroxylation of lysine into hydroxylysine in collagen. In individuals who suffer from a deficiency of this vitamin, the α-chains of the tropocollagen molecules are unable to form stable helices and the tropocollagen molecules are incapable of aggregating into fibrils. It first impacts connective tissues with a high turnover of collagen, along with the periodontal ligament and gingiva. Avitaminosis C is associated with the failure of wound healing or the rupture of capillaries because of intrinsic intercellular weakness with lack of connective tissue support of the capillary walls. Among the presenting features of scurvy, oral signs may be cardinal: Fetid odor and loosened teeth, gingivae are boggy, ulcerated and bleed with the interdental and marginal gingiva becoming bright red, smooth, swollen and shiny (LZG. 1984).

Clinical Implications of Periodontal Connective Tissue

Periodontal therapy has historically been directed primarily at the elimination of disease and the maintenance of a functional, healthy dentition and supporting tissues. Accordingly, the World Workshop in Periodontics 1989 has recommended the goals of periodontal therapy as immediate, ideal, pragmatic, and ultimate, mainly considering the disease status and patient's ability to maintain oral hygiene and comply with the periodontist's instructions.

While these goals still remain important, an acceptable esthetic outcome has been added as part of periodontal therapy in the last two decades. Patients are increasingly becoming conscious of a pleasing gingival display in addition to tooth form and color. Probably, one of the most common esthetic concerns associated with the periodontal tissues is gingival recession. Esthetics, progression of recession, hypersensitivity, or difficulties with oral hygiene may warrant the need to cover exposed roots. Esthetics plays a very important role on a person's psyche. Therefore, restoring the lost esthetics forms an important aspect of cosmetic surgery, which in turn improves the patient's appearance and self-esteem. Gingival recession or marginal soft tissue recession is the displacement of the gingival margin apical to the cementoenamel junction. Recession of gingival tissues from the root surfaces of teeth has long been a concern of many patients who feel that the "long-in-the-tooth" look is universally accepted as a sign of ageing and tooth loss (An, Dentistry, and Program 2009). Although gingival recession seldom results in tooth loss, its sequel, such as tooth hypersensitivity, root caries and esthetic concerns can be difficult to treat. The exposed root surfaces are also more prone to abrasion. Any one of these problems or a combination of these, along with patient's intense esthetic desire prompts the patient to seek treatment for gingival recession.

Mucogingival procedures are a form of periodontal reconstructive surgery. The primary objective of these procedures is to benefit periodontal health through the reconstruction of lost hard and soft tissues or by preventing further loss. They are also known as periodontal plastic surgical procedures which consist of a variety of procedures including root coverage, crown lengthening, vestibular deepening, papilla reconstruction, and ridge augmentation. It is one of the most common and accepted procedure for root coverage through a variety of gingival grafting techniques have been advocated to treat gingival recession namely lateral pedicle flaps, coronally positioned flaps, free gingival grafts, connective tissue grafts, and guided tissue regeneration. Harmony between hard and soft tissue morphologies is essential for form, function, and a good esthetic outlook. Replacement grafts for correction of soft tissue defects around the teeth have become important to periodontal plastic and implant surgical procedures.

Among many of surgical techniques and graft materials reported in the literature, the subepithelial connective tissue graft (SCTG) has gained wide popularity and acceptance due its various benefits lesser postoperative complication. The maximum amount of SCTG can be harvested from a U-shaped palatal vault. Soft tissues that extend about 2-4 mm from the cementoenamel junction of maxillary posterior teeth contain a dense lamina propria; beyond this region, glandular structures and submucosa are encountered (Karthikeyan et al. 2016). SCTGs from the posterior palate are usually denser but limited in size, whereas SCTGs from the anterior palate are loose in consistency but can be larger. Clinical experience recommends that SCTGs be harvested from the posterior part of the palate when better volume stability over time is desirable, such as in soft tissue augmentation procedures. On the other hand, this type of graft seems to be more sensitive to the local blood supply for its revascularization. SCTG promoted a more favorable increase in keratinized tissue. Both techniques for treatment of gingival recession lead to favorable and long-term stable results.

TECHNIQUES FOR HARVESTING A SUBEPITHELIAL CONNECTIVE TISSUE GRAFT (SCTG) FROM THE PALATE

Edel (1974) first described the technique of harvesting SCTGs from the palate to increase the width of the attached gingiva. He suggested to harvest tissue from the palatal mucosa, but later areas, such as the maxillary tuberosity, were also utilized. (Figure 14)

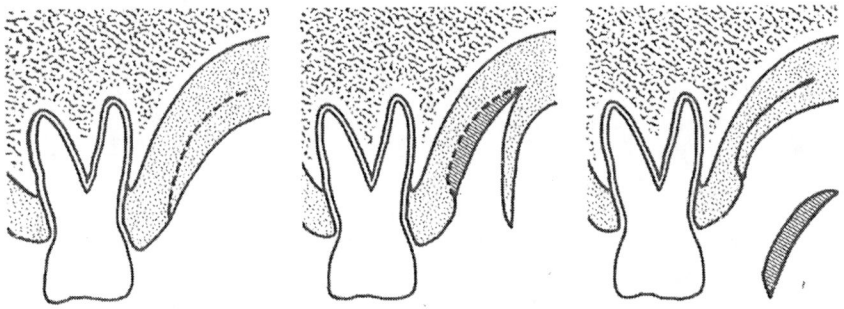

Figure 14. A partial thickness flap is raised and the connective tissue graft is taken from below the palatal surface. The flap is suture back.

Langer and Calagna (1980) proposed a variant for CTG procedure many modifications have been presented for harvesting the graft from donor as well as its use at the recipient site. Over time, the SCTG technique has produced the most predictable results for obtaining root coverage.

He conducted a study for predictability of SCTG in obtaining stable RC for a long time was especially verified in several studies using different periods of evaluation. Root coverage stability of the subepithelial connective tissue graft was considered to be stable.

Roman et al. (2013) reported the treatment of gingival recessions with a connective tissue graft and coronally advanced flap. The clinical and histological results were observed after 12 months. Clinically, the grafted tissues seemed to be attached to the root surfaces, and the histological results indicated that the healing resulted in a long connective tissue attachment, which was shown to be stable over time. (Figure 15)

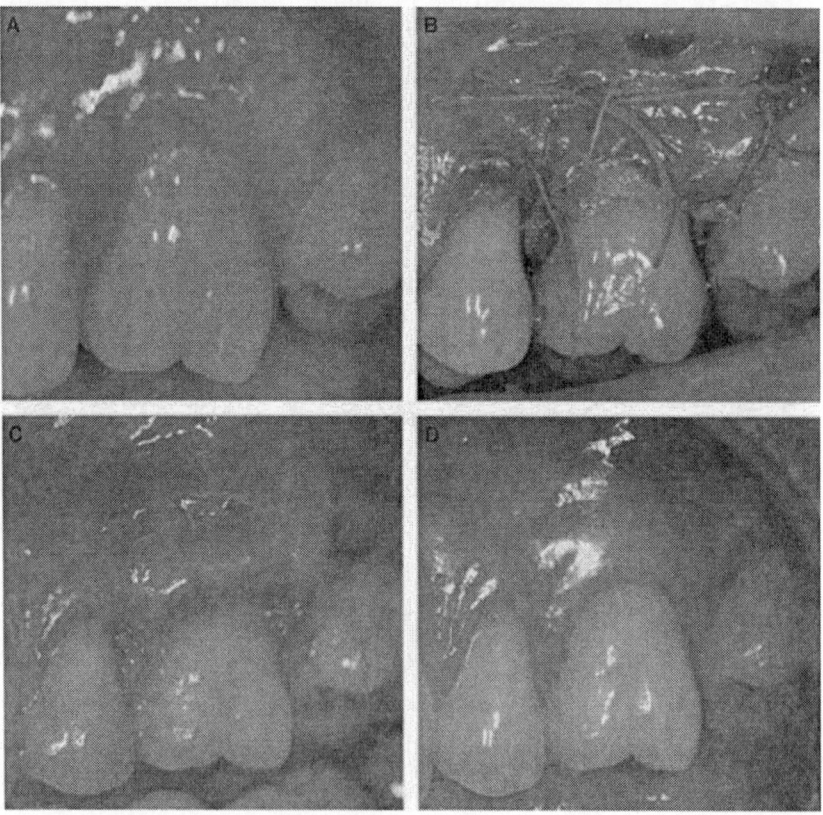

Figure 15. Connective tissue graft done by Roman et al. technique.

Trapdoor Technique (Nelson 1987)

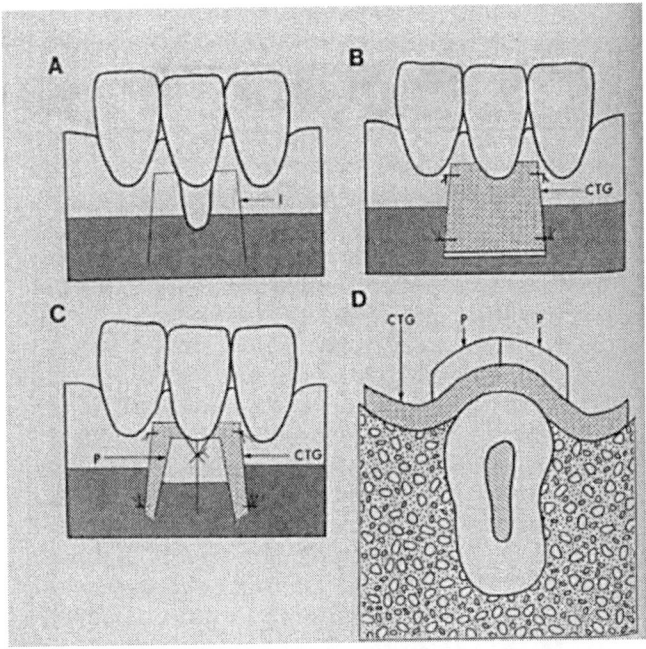

Figure 16. Incisions (I) are made to include as much of the inter-dental papilla as possible without affecting the adjacent teeth. Full thickness flaps are reflected. B. Following root planing a connective tissue graft (CTG) is sutured with resorbable sutures. The connective tissue graft should cover the cemento-enamel junction of the tooth as sutured together over the free connective tissue graft (CTG). They well as the donor pedicle sites. C. The interdental pedicles (P) are should cover the a vascular part of the free connective tissue graft which overlies the denuded root surface. D. A cross section of the sub-pedicle suturing the pedicles (P) over the affected root, plasmatic circulation covering the denuded root as well as the donor pedicle sites. By connective tissue graft shows the free connective tissue graft (CTG) will be supplied to the free connective tissue graft below.

A variant to conventional technique, this technique uses palatal portion opposite to the molars is selected for harvesting the graft. A primary incision is made along the long axis of the teeth, near the gingival margin. A total of 1 horizontal and 2 vertical incisions are made, the flap is raised, and the graft is harvested. The undersurface of an edentulous region can also be used for harvesting the graft. Complete wound closure is achieved.

- *Advantages:* Visibility and accessibility is better than conventional technique. Complete wound closure is obtained. Healing is by primary intention
- *Disadvantages:* More number of sutures are required and the site is more prone to slough formation due to compromised blood supply. (Fig 16, 17)

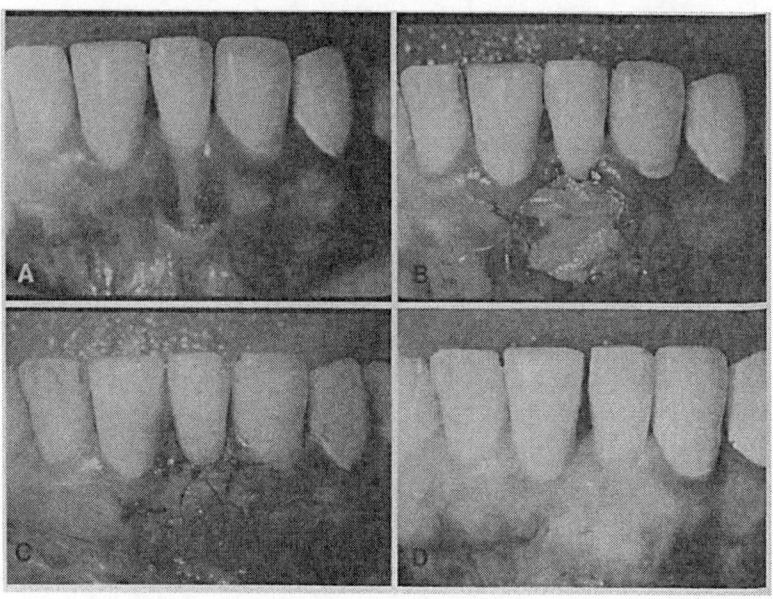

Figure 17. Step wise procedure done by trapdoor technique.

Broome and Taggart (1976) trapdoor using Brasher-Rees knife 1976:

- *Advantages:* Brasher-Rees knife is a specialized equipment for procedure. It allows wider base minimizes the postoperative discomfort and reduces healing time, use leads to adequate amount of graft harvest.
- *Disadvantages:* Vertical incisions may compromise blood supply and lead to sloughing; special armamentarium required. (Figure 18, 19, 20)

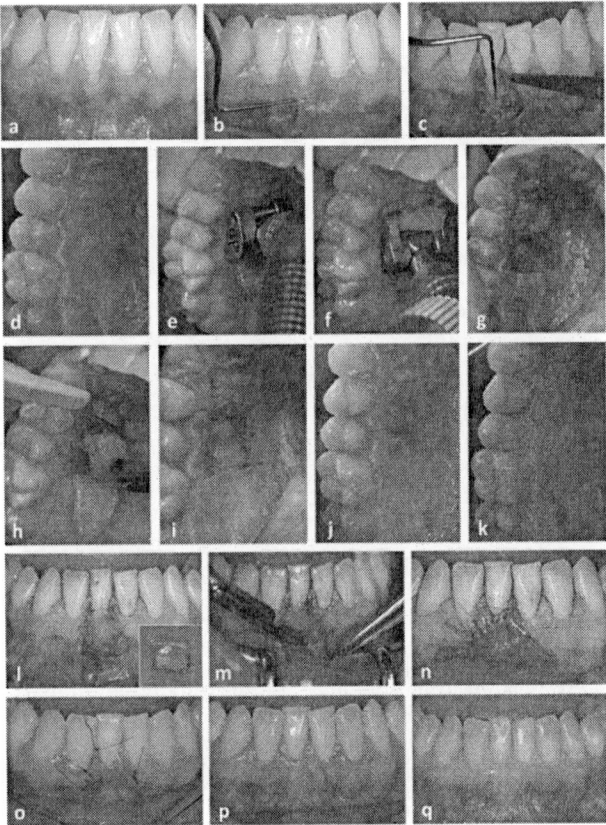

Figure 18. Stepwise photographs of broome and taggart technique.

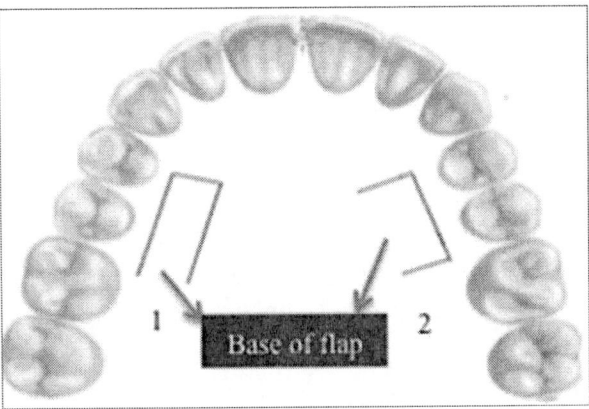

Figure 19. Borders for the broome taggart technique.

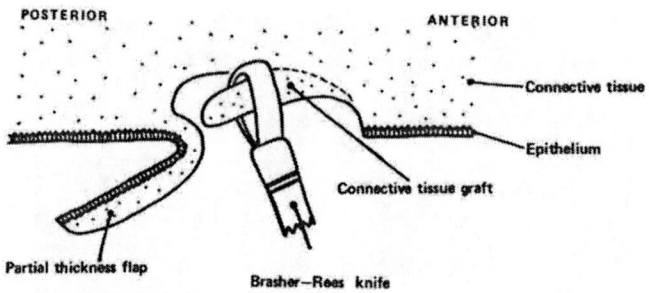

Figure 20. Brasher- Rees knife.

Technique By Langer and Calagna (1980) and Lourenço et al. (2007)

A horizontal bevel incision is made on the palate 1 mm apical to the free gingival margin of the posterior teeth. This is followed by vertical incisions at either end, and the graft is harvested from the palatal side. In the presence of periodontal pockets, an internal bevel flap is created for pocket elimination. Connective tissue and epithelium are recovered from the excised pocket wall. The band of epithelium in the harvested tissue is discarded, while connective tissue is retained. A rectangular design, with 2 horizontal and 2 vertical incisions, results in an SCTG with an epithelial collar of 1.5-2.0 mm in width. The technique overcame multiple limitations associated with free gingival graft techniques, including poor esthetic integration, unsatisfactory quantitative insufficient augmentation volume and, surface texture, and color; scarring.

Advantage: There is decreased tendency for graft shrinkage. There is epithelium band along with graft is present to provide smoother junction with the existing epithelium, bi-laminar blood supply, epithelium band along with graft to provide smoother junction with the existing epithelium.

Disadvantage: On donor site complete wound closure is not obtained and the vertical incisions may compromise blood supply. Vertical incisions may compromise blood supply, on donor site, at times complete wound closure is not obtained; CTG with parts of the epithelium leaves an uncovered part of the donor area that has to heal by secondary intention. Complete closure of the donor site is not seen because of the rigidity of the palatal mucosa.

Envelope Technique (Raetzke 1985)

This technique employs no vertical incisions but 2 converging horizontal, crescent-shaped incisions that intersect deep within the palate, producing a wedge of SCTG with an epithelial collar. (Figure 21-23)

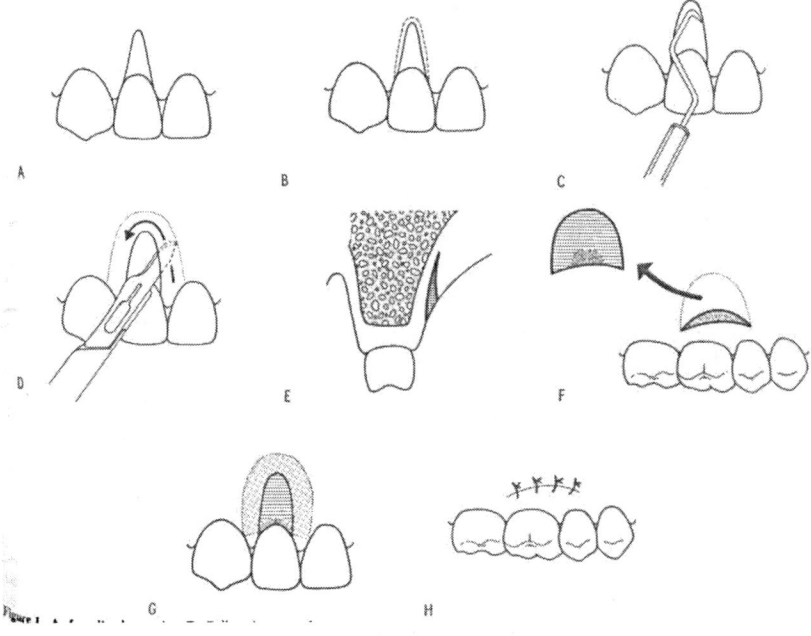

Figure 21. A. Localized recession. B. Collar of marginal tissue excised. C. Root is debrided and planed. D. Undermining partial thickness incision creating "envelope." E. Sagittal view of palatal incisions. F. Connective tissue wedge is removed. Epithelium is excised except for the part comes to lie over the exposed root. G. Graft placed in the envelope completely covers the formerly denuded root surface. H. Wound edges adapted and sutured.

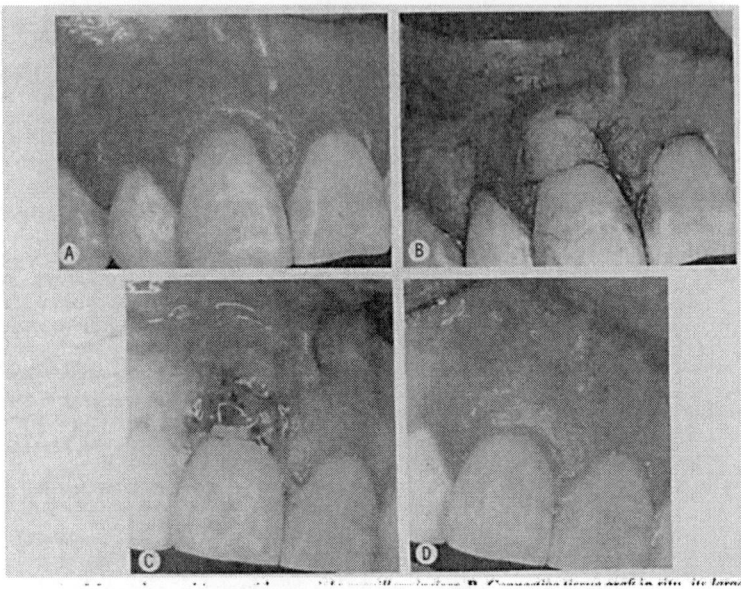

Figure 22. A. Recession 2.5 mm deep andò mm wide over right maxillary incisor. B, Connective tissue graft in situ, its larger part situated in the envelope. Appearance 1 week after surgery, Capillaries can be seen within the graft. Rests of epithelium are adherent. D. Appearance 2 months after surgery. Complete coverage of formerly denuded root surface. Clinical sulcus depth is 1 mm.

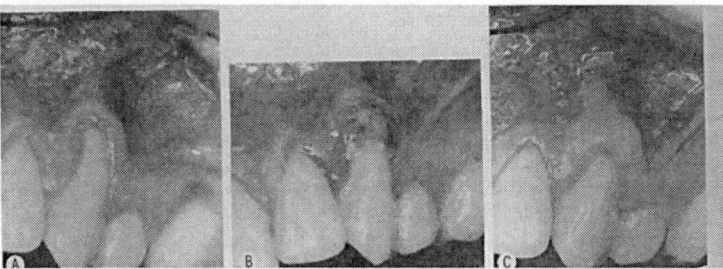

Figure 23. A. Recession 4 mm deep and 3 mm wide over left maxillary canine. B. Appearance 1 week after surgery. Again, capillaries can be seen within the graft. C. 8 months after surgery. Complete coverage has been obtained. A wide zone of keratinized gingiva has formed. Clinical sulcus depth is 1 mm.

- *Advantage:* Suitable for single tooth recession defect, minor wound at donor site, healing by primary intention, no vertical incisions.

- *Disadvantage:* Donor tissue area from where epithelial band was obtained might heal due to secondary intention. Cannot be used in patients with a more generalized periodontal recession because the availability of donor tissue obtained is limited, particularly in patients with thin palatal mucosa.

Double-Blade Knife Technique (Harris 1992, 1994)

A graft knife is used to elevate a split-thickness flap, which is attached distally to the palate in this modification of the original trapdoor technique. At the distal edge of the connective tissue, the knife is then pulled mesially under the trapdoor flap to elevate a SCTG. Using a Harris double-bladed graft knife, an instrument with two blades placed 1.5 mm apart, will simplify the technique. Two methods (parallel blade technique and knife technique)

- *Advantage:* dense connective tissue graft is obtained uniformly.
- *Disadvantage:* CTG leaves an exposed portion of the donor with portions of the epithelium

Single Incision Technique (Hürzeler & Weng 1999)

On the palate, 2 mm from marginal gingiva, a single horizontal incision is made. First the knife is angled to 90 degrees, then to weaken the flap is angled to 135 degrees. The SCTG is extracted by making both sides of the exposed SCTG incision into the bone. This method has several advantages: preventing sloughing of the epithelium due to an undesirable relationship between the base of the flap and the duration of the pedicle, increasing postoperative healing and reducing patient morbidity. (Figure 24)

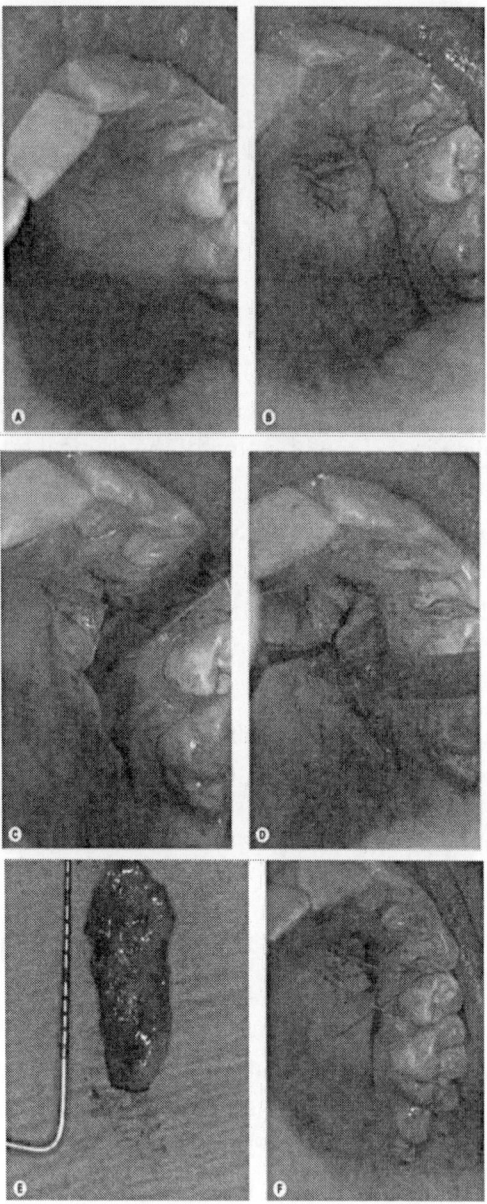

Figure 24. A. Palatal site UL346. B. Superficial palatal incision 2–3 mm below the gingival margin. C. Vertical incision running parallel to the palate splitting the palatal flap from the connective tissue. D. The connective tissue is raised off the periosteum. E. The harvested connective tissue graft. F. Compressive sutures to stabilize the flap to the palate bone.

- *Advantage:* first single-incision technique; primary purpose healing; no vertical incisions, therefore no blood supply compromised; reduced number of sutures; technique is applicable for different anatomic situations of the palatal vault.
- *Disadvantage:* Reduced visibility as single incision; first incision full thickness to bone, so bleeding can jeopardize accessibility and visibility.

Method of Double-Incision (Bruno 1994)

The first incision is made perpendicular to the teeth's long axis, about 2-3 mm apical to the maxillary teeth's gingival edge, falling short of the bone.

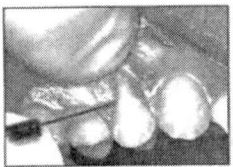
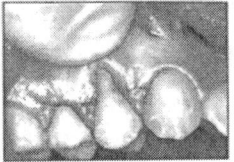
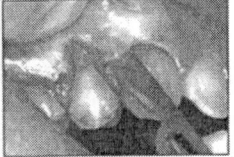

Figure 25. Initial horizontal right-angle incision is mode into the papillae with a 12B surgical blade. The initial incision is made at or coronal to the CEJ of the tooth with the exposed toot surface. Sharp dissection is accomplished with a #15 surgical blade to create a partial-thickness flap.

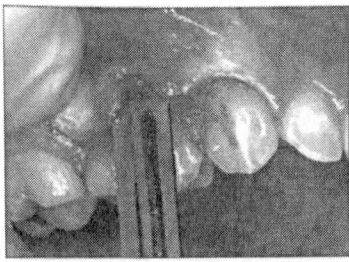
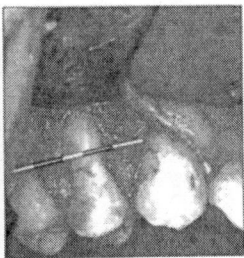

Figure 26. The incision is extended apically into the muco-buccal fold well beyond the muco-gingival junction. A periodontal probe is used to obtain the approximate width of the donor tissue that will be required for the recipient site. Note the extent of the hidden recession that is revealed.

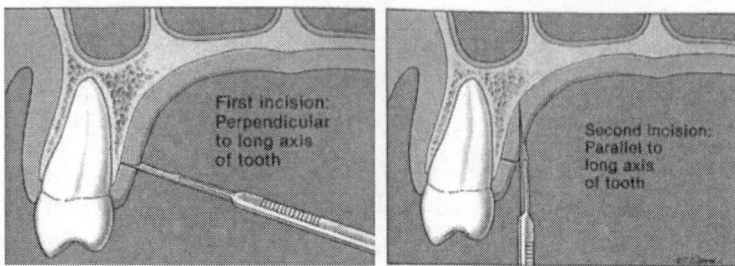

Figure 27. The first incision at the donor site on the palate is made approximately 2 to 3 mm apical to the gingival margins of the teeth. The second incision at the donor site is made 1 to 2 mm apical to the first incision. The more apical the incision, the thicker the donor tissue will be.

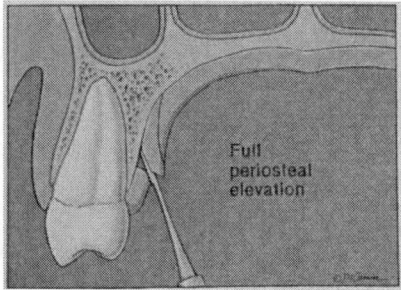

Figure 28. A small periosteal elevator is used to raise o full-thickness connective-tissue flap.

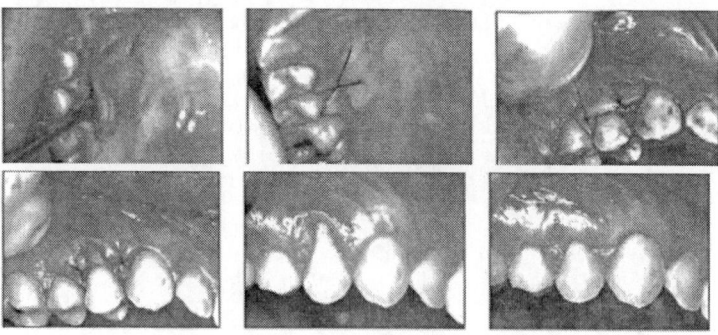

Figure 29. Note the convergence of the incisions at their mesial and distal borders. The palatal wound is approximated with a crossed horizontal suspension suture. The donor connective tissue is stabilized with Interrupted sutures. In this case, a 1-mm band of epithelium is retained at the coronal margin at the graft. The overlying partial-thickness flap is replaced with Interrupted sutures into the papillae. Preoperative view. Two-month postoperative view.

The second incision is made parallel to the teeth's long axis, but 1-2 mm apical to the first incision. A small periosteal elevator is used to lift a full thickness periosteal SCTG (double incision) (Figure 25-29)

- *Advantage:* no vertical incisions, so no impaired blood supply and reduced patient pain during healing time, preservation of vascular periosteum on the donor tissue can provide increased circulation to the graft; more consistent thickness of the palatal flap so less risk of sloughing.
- *Disadvantage:* No vertical incisions, so the procedure is somewhat difficult due to limited access; also due to the stiffness of the palatal masticatory mucosa, which does not allow the donor site to be completely closed, part of the donor site may be cured by secondary intention.(Fig 25,26)

Technique By Lorenzana and Allen (2000)

This approach is similar to the technique defined by Hürzeler & Weng, except that vertical (mesial and distal) and medial incisions are not made to relieve the graft. Instead, careful handling of the graft is required with corn suture pinions or other delicate tissue forceps. Care must be taken to prevent the graft from being squeezed or teared.

- *Advantage:* Healing by primary intention; it is possible to obtain large amounts of graft with accelerated healing and minimal patient pain.
- *Disadvantage:* Since no vertical incisions are used, a sufficient extension of the first horizontal incision is required to obtain the desired dimensions of the graft.

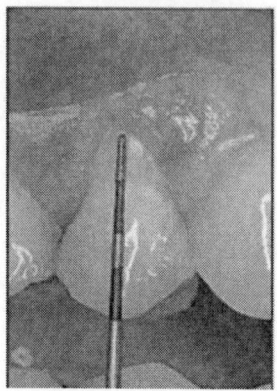
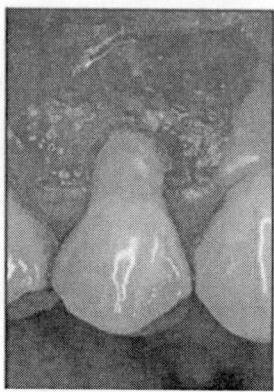

Figure 30. Maxillary right second premolar with a 4-mm Miller Class I recession. Split-thickness recipient bed preparations.

A single access incision is applied to the bone adjacent to the surface of the palatal tissue. A split-thickness dissection is made in conjunction with the long axis of the teeth through this incision to dissect the graft from the underlying bone and superficial tissues. There is no blunt periosteal elevator dissection, leaving the periosteum on the surface of the bone. This method helps to shape granulation tissue in the wound and speeds up the palatal donor site's repair. (Fig 30-34)

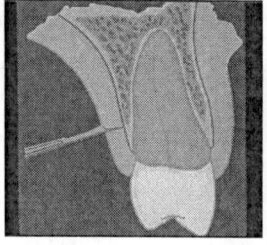
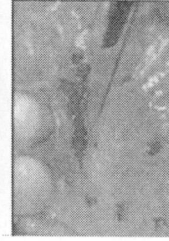
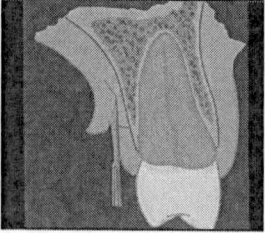

Figure 31. Initial incision is made with # 15 blade oriented perpendicular to the tissue surface. Single palatal incision. Split-thickness dissection is made parallel to the long axis of the teeth, leaving the graft attached to the underlying bone with adequate thickness of the overlying palatal flap.

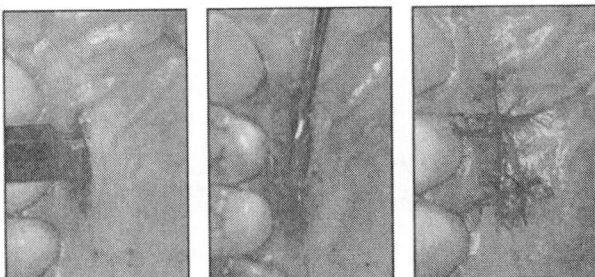

Figure 32. Split-thickness dissection. Atraumatic graft elevation using a Molt periosteal elevator. Primary closure of donor site is achieved with # 5.0 chromic gut sutures.

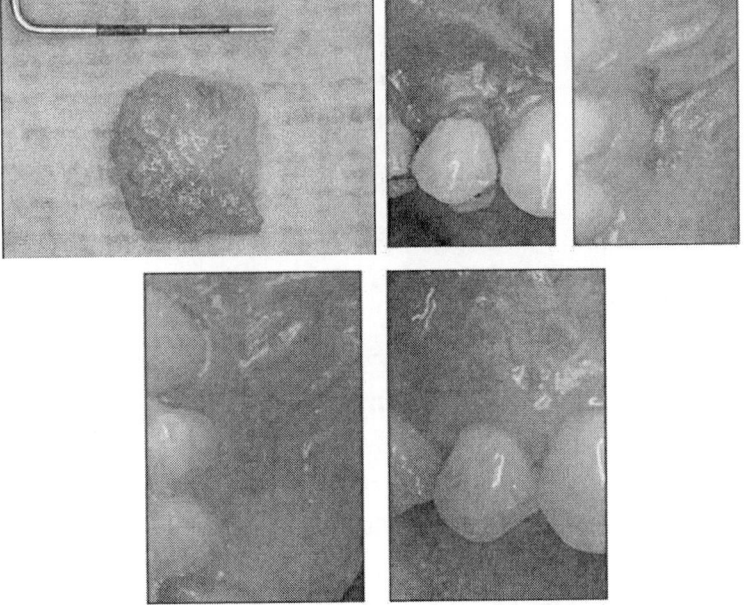

Figure 33. Harvested connective tissue graft (periosteum side). Final suturing of grafted site. Healing at 5 days following graft harvesting. Healing at 2 weeks. Note accelerated healing response of the palatal wound. After 15 months, 100% root coverage is maintained. Single incision technique (Del Pizzo et al. 2002)

- *Advantage:* reduced number of incisions; periosteum was not removed along with connective tissue as it helps in the formation of granulated tissue and accelerates the healing of wounds.
- *Disadvantage*: Reduced visibility.

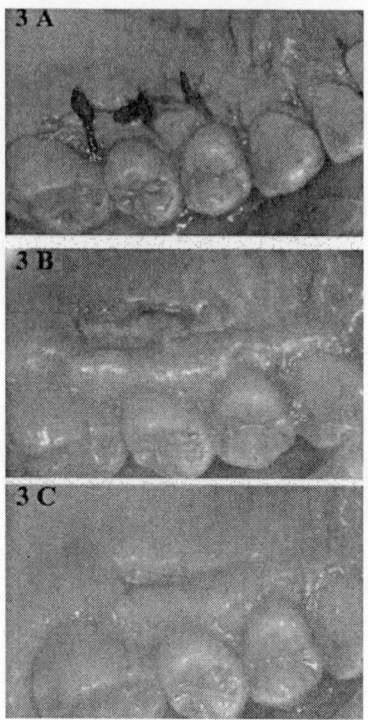

Figure 34. A. Postsurgery. B. 1st week follow-up visit. C. 2nd week follow-up visit.

Technique By Zucchelli et al. (2010)

- *Advantage:* it is possible to obtain FGG in situations where there are undesirable palatal anatomical conditions that can be extraorally deepened.
- *Disadvantage:* The donor site heals by secondary intention.

Technique of Extended Mesh (Deniz Çetiner 2004)

- *Advantage:* Treatment with minimal donor tissue in one operation for multiple recession defects.

- *Disadvantage:* Thick grafting is important and it is not always possible to obtain an intact and thick graft; it could result in the graft being perforated/separated. (Figure 35)

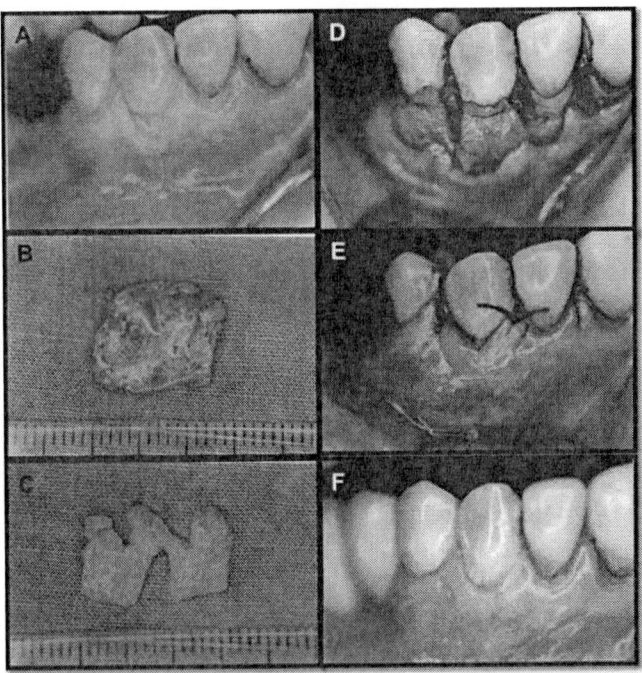

Figure 35. Step-Wise Technique of harvesting connective tissue graft By Deniz Centiner method.

Technique By Bosco and Bosco (2007)

From the sides of a 1.5-mm incision, a split-thickness flap is raised to hold the periosteum intact. A dense graft is collected, composed of epithelium and connective tissue. The graft is put and bisected on a sterile cloth. One of the resulting grafts is epithelium with connective tissue, while the other is connective tissue only. On the donor site, the epithelial graft is repositioned as a free gingival graft and parodontal dressing is applied with or without a suture for compression. (Figure 36)

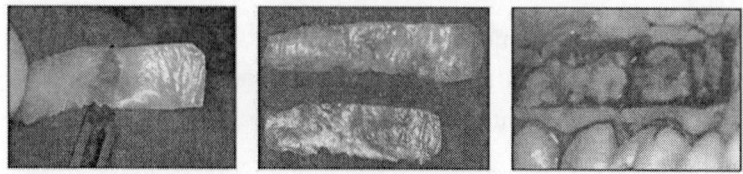

Figure 36. Removal of the external layer of the graft. View of the connective tissue and epithelialized grafts. The epithelialized graft is repositioned at the donor site and secured with compression.

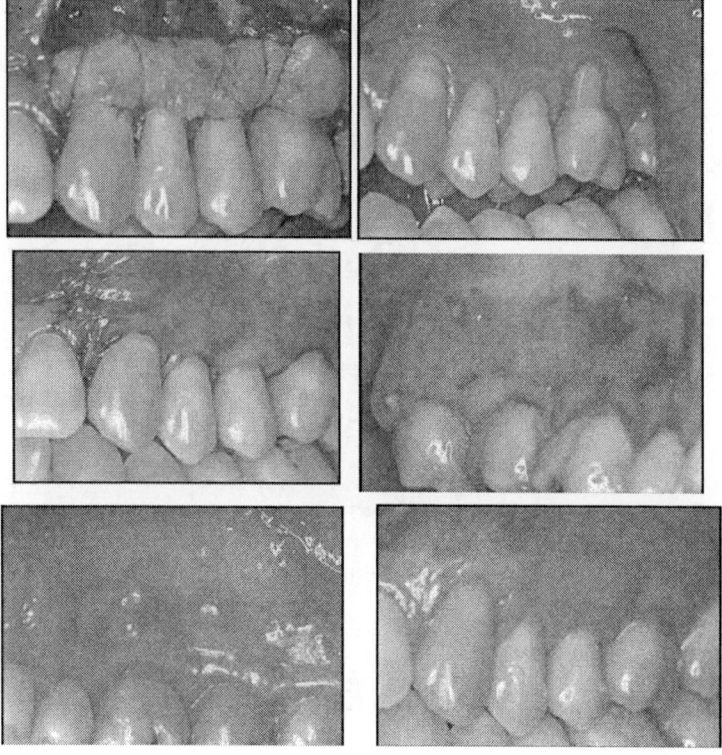

Figure 37.1. Preoperative view of the Miller Class I gingival recessions on the buccal of the canine and first and second premolars and Miller Class II recession on the mesiobuccal root of the first molar. A connective tissue graft is sutured over the recession defects. The flap is positioned coronally and sutured, completely covering the graft and the denuded root surfaces. Sites at 10 days postoperative. The palate is completely epithelialized and is in the maturation stage. Patient at 20 days postoperative (mirror view). The donor area is completely healed. Six months postoperative. Complete coverage of the areas of recession is apparent.

- *Advantage:* Procurement of tissue from shallow palate or palate with thin mucosa; prevents damage to palate vessels; enables graft extraction with limited adipose and glandular tissue of submucosa.
- *Disadvantage:* This procedure is daunting for clinicians as it is often difficult to bisect a thin FGG successfully; it is not always possible to obtain an intact and dense graft; it could lead to unnecessary graft perforation.

Technique By Ribeiro et al. and Pontes et al. (2008)

The SCTG is harvested using a single-incision technique with full thickness so that it can be broken cross-sectionally. Nevertheless, the graft is not completely divided into 2 parts; thus, it is nearly twice the length of the original graft and is about 1.5 mm thick (split CTG technique) (Figure 37, 38)

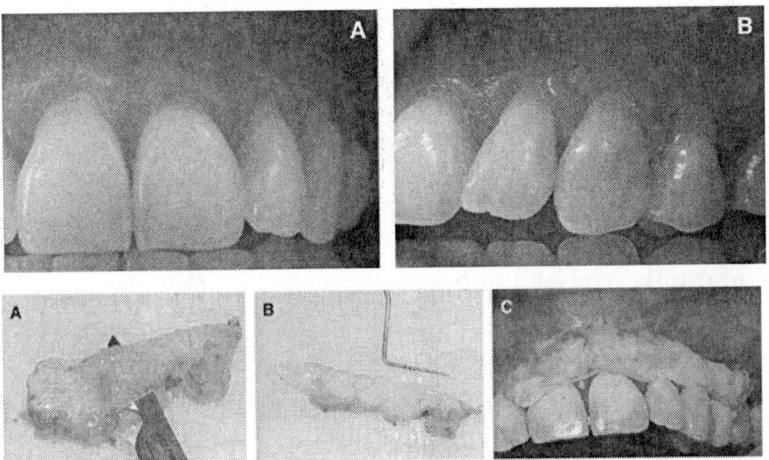

Figure 37.

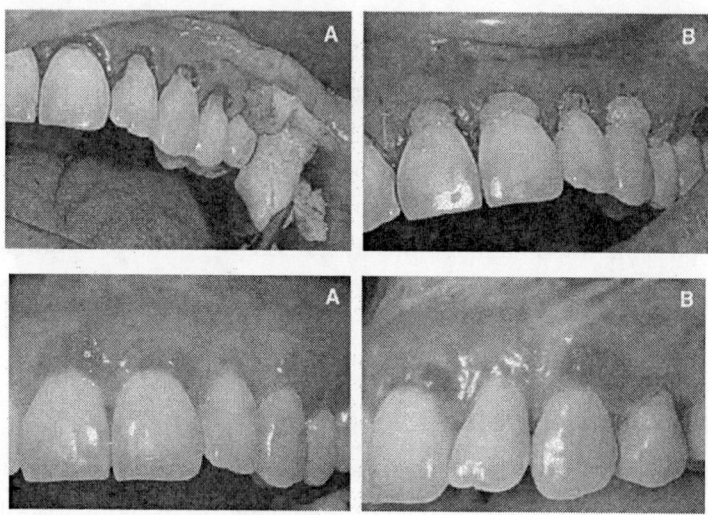

Figure 38. Stepwise procedure of connective tissue graft by Ribeirio et al. technique.

- *Advantage:* Graft width is obtained approximately twice the original graft length and acceptable thickness.
- *Disadvantage:* Practice is challenging in cases where there is inadequate palatal tissue thickness leading to graft perforation; It is often difficult to bisect a thin graft successfully; It is not always possible to obtain an intact and dense graft.

Technique By McLeod and Elio Reyes (2009) (Figure 39-42)

In order to epithelialize the palatal donor site from the mesial side of the canine to the distal part of the first molar, a sharp back-action periodontal chisel is used. The SCTG is harvested with a surgical blade after deep-hyalinization in the manner used to harvest a traditional free gingival graft.

- *Advantage:* Simple technique; partial palatal de-epithelialization leads to procurement of a thin, uniform, and abundant connective tissue graft from the palate to treat multiple areas of gingival

recession; eliminates the challenges of bisecting the thin graft; suturing not required; tissue harvested is usually adequate to treat recession in an entire arch with excess tissue remaining, depending on the size of the patient's palate; tissue harvested is firmer than conventional CTG so easy to handle and less slippery.
- *Disadvantage:* As the harvest approaches the palatal midline, it is important to adhere to the recommended measurement because the mucosal tissue in the midline is thinner and the collateral blood vessels in the area may lead to abundant bleeding.

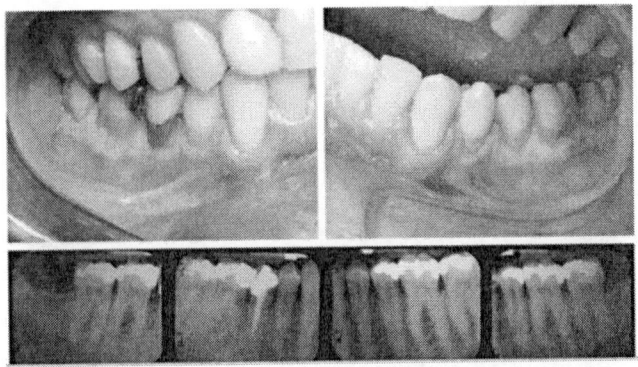

Figure 39. Initial view of teeth #18 through #22 (top left) and #27 through #31 (top right) showing generalized gingival recession. Periapical radiographs of mandibular right (two bottom left radiographs) and left posterior teeth (two bottom right radiographs) showing slight interproximal bone loss.

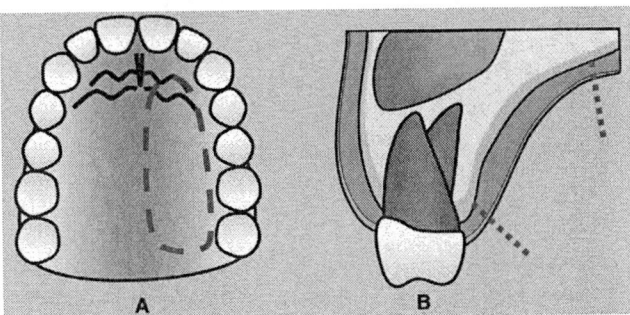

Figure 40. The simple harvesting technique for connective tissue graft; the broken lines represent the limits for tissue procurement. A) Occlusal view. B) Frontal view.

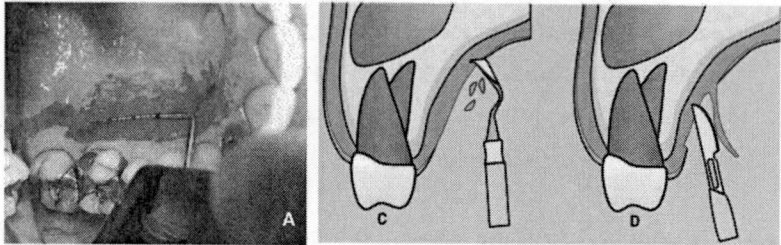

Figure 41. Palatal wound after deepithelialization. B) Photomicrograph of connective tissue showing remnants of the basal layer of the palatal epithelium (hematoxylin and eosin; original magnification, x 10. C) Donor site deepithelialized with a sharp back-action surgical periodontal chisel. D) Procurement of thin connective tissue graft using a surgical knife with a #15C blade.

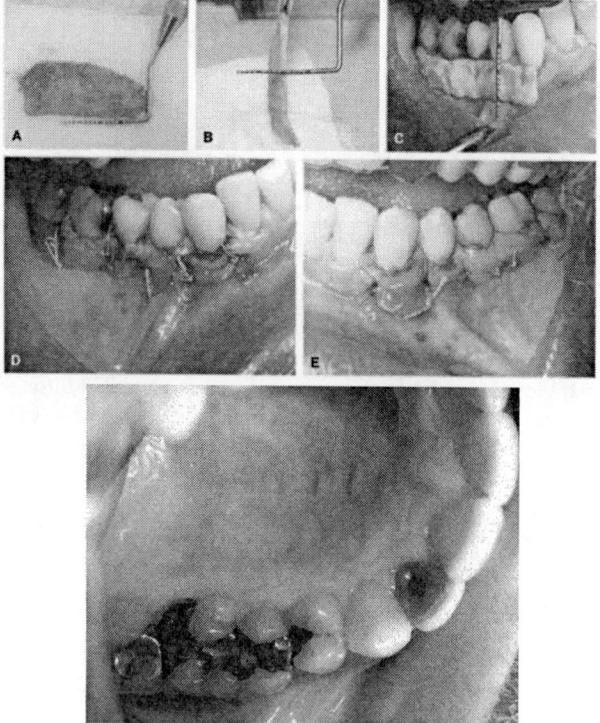

Figure 42. Length and width of the connective tissue graft. B) Thickness of the graft as demonstrated using a University of North Carolina periodontal probe. C) Width of the connective tissue graft for teeth #27 through #31. Simple mattress suturing of connective tissue graft and overlying mucosa on right (D) and left (E) sides.

Technique By Stimmelmayr M, Allen EP, Reichert TE (2010) (Epithelized-subepithelial Connective Tissue Graft)

- *Advantage*: Potential reduction of graft necrosis
- *Disadvantage:* Increased morbidity of the donor site due to secondary healing in the open wound region.

Ramakrishnan, Kaur, and Aggarwal (2011) (Epithelial Embossed Connective Tissue Graft 2011)

- *Advantage*: Preserved embossed epithelium at the coronal boundary of the subepithelial connective tissue graft that fits exactly the defect to be treated.
- *Disadvantage:* Portion of the donor site is left open for healing by secondary intention.

Technique By Kumar et al. (2013)

- *Advantages:* First incision is partial thickness so less bleeding is encountered; improved visibility, better estimate of the size of the connective tissue graft and better control of the incisions as there are no random angulations to be followed; new AVS instrument and Barraquer cataract knife are useful to overcome the difficulties faced by operators in making medial and vertical incisions respectively; reduced number of sutures compared to conventional techniques
- *Disadvantages:* Special armamentarium required; difficult to execute for new clinicians.

Modified Single Incision Technique (Reino 2013)

- *Advantages:* More accurate control of the graft thickness; periosteum left on donor bone to decrease patient discomfort or morbidity; healing by primary intention.
- *Disadvantages:* Technique might be difficult to execute for new clinicians as raised full-thickness flap was dissected to separate a partial-thickness connective tissue flap. (Figure 43, 44)

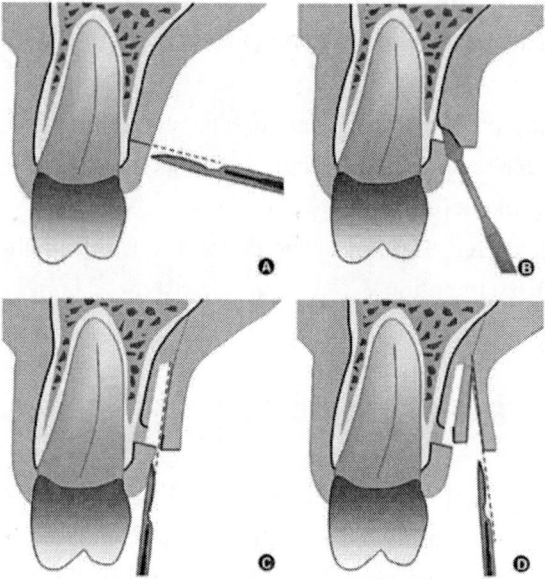

Figure 43. Schematic illustration of the new modification for the single incision palatal harvest technique. A: Incision perpendicular to the palatal tissue until reaching the bone in a horizontal direction. B: Elevation of 1 to 2 mm of a full thicknessflap. C: Dissection of the partial thickness flap. D: Graft harvesting from the flap.

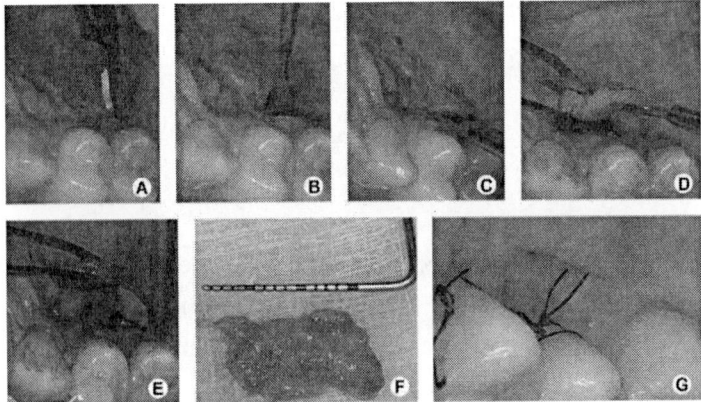

Figure 44. Surgery at the recipient site. A: Preoperative multiple gingival recession. B: Oblique incisions. C: SCTG fixed at the recipient site. D: Sutures. E: Postoperative image of the treated area after 6 months.

Technique By Aguirre-Zorzano et al.(2017)

- *Advantages:* Minimizes the occurrence of postoperative complications as compared to trapdoor technique.
- *Disadvantages:* Demanding technique in terms of the operator's skills as compared to trapdoor technique.

Controlled Palatal Harvest Technique (Bhatavadekar and Gharpure 2018)

- *Advantages:* Highly predictable procedure in ensuring adequate graft and flap thickness, ability to obtain uniform graft and flap thickness, and less chance of leaving behind a thin flap for closure at the donor site thereby minimizing necrosis and flap sloughing and improving grafting success.
- *Disadvantages:* Technique sensitive and dependent on the thickness of the palatal mucosa. In cases with thin mucosa, there is a chance of perforation of the flap while obtaining the graft; harvest procedure is done from a relatively mobile flap; as with

any incision perpendicular to the blood supply, increased bleeding is possible.

CLINICAL USES OF TISSUE GRAFT PROCEDURES

Various soft tissue graft procedures namely pedicle soft tissue graft, autogenous connective tissue Graft, non-Autogenous connective tissue Graft and combined connective tissue and double pedicle Graft procedures are indicated for the following:

- When there is less than 2 mm of attached gingiva
- Hypersensitivity associated with recession
- chronic inflammation and recession
- teeth with subgingival restorations
- ridge augmentation
- correct fit of prosthesis by increasing vestibular depth in abutment teeth widen zone of attached gingiva
- clefting of gingiva
- Surgical Periodontics: Regenerative Procedures
- Surgical Periodontics: Resective Procedures
- Treatment of soft tissue recession at implant site
- Augmentation of the width of keratinized gingival
- Preservation of the ridge with implant and fixed partial dentures procedure
- Augmentation of gingival thickness following or prior to orthodontic therapy
- Augmentation of gingival thickness following or prior to restorative therapy
- Reconstruction of soft tissue and coverage of maxillary defects
- interdental papilla reconstruction
- periimplantitis tissues correction
- Closure of defects following apicoectomy

- Intraosseous subperiosteal connective tissue graft for reduction of pockets and management of furcations as combined procedures
- Correction of localized gingival pigmentation
- Masking of visible implant components
- Correct discrepancy of gingival thickness prior to orthodontic therapy
- Correct discrepancy of gingival thickness following or prior to restorative therapy
- Reconstruction of soft tissue and coverage of maxillary defects
- Surgical reconstruction of interdental papilla
- Management of peri-implant tissues
- Closure of defects following apicoectomy
- Management of grade II furcations defects
- Depigmentation of gingival soft tissue
- Masking of discolored roots or visible implant components
- Preservation of the ridge with implant and fixed partial dentures procedure

Autogenous connective tissue graft autogenous connective tissue procedures are not indicated for the following:

- Thin bony plates
- Medically compromised patients
- Autogenous connective tissue Graft is not indicated when there is a broad, shallow palatal donor site, or excessively glandular or fatty submucosal tissue in donor site

Benefits of Subepithelial Connective Tissue Grafts (Karthikeyan et al. 2016)

- Dual blood supply.
- Esthetic matching of color matching around the recipient site and better topograph

- Healing of donor site occurs by primary intention thus no scarring.
- greater predictability of outcome
- Minimal discomfort to the patient and the healing is uneventful.

POTENTIAL COMPLICATIONS OF THE SUBEPITHELIAL CONNECTIVE TISSUE GRAFT

Donor Site Complications

- Necrosis of graft and palatal site complications
- Pain and excessive blood loss
- Prolonged uneasyness
- Increased chances of infection at donor site
- loss of sensation in palate in rare cases

Recipient Site Complications

- Postsurgical swelling and ecchymosis
- External root resorption
- formation of gingival cysts
- soft tissue abscess formation of gingiva
- Exostosis
- Graft loss
- Epithelial cell discharge
- Reaction to suture material
- Gingival cul-de-sac defects
- Suturing under tension may lead to obliteration of microcirculation

Cause of Failure to Provide Root Coverage

- Insufficient height of interdental bone
- Reflection of all interdental papilla
- Horizontal incision placed apical to cementoenamel junction
- Flap penetration
- Graft that is too thick or too thin
- Tension in graft
- Ineffective postsurgical biofilm control during healing
- Inadequate height and thickness of keratinized tissue

CONCLUSION

Connective tissue is an important tissue of the body and originates from the mesenchyme that is the middle layer of the embryonic germ layer. Various types of cells are the part of connective tissue.

Periodontal disease starts early in life and can lead to dire consequences, such as gingival recession, loss of involved teeth, and consequently, alveolar ridge defects. A number of procedures have been used to regenerate supporting tooth structures. Among them, the subepithelial connective tissue graft (SCTG) has been regarded as a reliable and predictable procedure that provides a satisfactory esthetic outcome, making it a popular alternative for clinicians. Major advantages of the SCTG are that it is inexpensive, versatile, and easily available; it provides successful outcomes; it is less invasive than other autogenous harvesting techniques; and it has a shorter healing period. Over the last few years, the SCTG has become the backbone of various treatment options for gingival recession coverage, existing or impending ridge deficiencies, management of peri implant tissue anomalies, and treatment of furcation involvement and thin gingiva. Currently, the SCTG is considered the gold standard for soft tissue correction and augmentation surgeries.

REFERENCES

Adams, D, Carney JS, Dicks DA. 1973. "Pregnancy Gingivitis: A Survey of 100 Antenatal Patients." *J Dent Res* 2: 106–10.

Aguirre-Zorzano, Luis Antonio, Ana M. García De La Fuente, Ruth Estefanía-Fresco, and Xabier Marichalar-Mendía. 2017. "Complications of Harvesting a Connective Tissue Graft from the Palate. A Retrospective Study and Description of a New Technique." *Journal of Clinical and Experimental Dentistry* 9 (12): e1439–45. https://doi.org/10.4317/jced.54337.

Alberts, B, Johnson A, Lewis J, Raff M, Roberts K, Walter P. 2002. Fibroblasts and Their Transformations: The Connective-Tissue Cell Family. InMolecular Biology of the Cell. *In Molecular Biology of the Cell.* 4th Edition.

Al-Jobeir, Asma. 2006. "Hereditary Epidermolysis Bullosa: Report of Two Cases." *Saudi Dental Journal* 18 (3): 155–61.

Al-Mulla, Maysah Faisal. 2013. "Marfan Syndrome : A Case Study." *International Jornal of Scientific Sudy* 1 (1): 38–47.

An, Gregory, Geriatric Dentistry, and Fellowship Program. 2009. "Normal Aging of Teeth." *Geriatrics and Ageing* 12 (10): 513–17.

Anonymous. n.d. "Oral Reactions to Non-Steroidal Antiinflammatory Drugs." *Repr Fr Adverse Drug Reactions Advisory Committee Bulletin,Assoc, Aust Dent Bull, News* 154: 17.

Bancroft, JD, Gamble M, Editors. n.d. *Theory and Practice of Histological Techniques.*

Banold I'M. 1989. "Regulation of Human Gingival Fibroblast Growth and Synthetic Activity by Cyclosporine-A in v i M." *J Periodontal Res.* 24: 314-21.

Bartold, PM, Narayan AS. 1988. *Biology of the Periodontal Connective Tissues. Quintessence Publishing (IL).*

Bartold, PM. 1987. "Proteoglycans of the Periodontium: Structure, Role and Function." *J. Periodont Res.* 22: 431–44.

Bartold, PM. 1992. "Distribution of Chondroitin Sulfate and Dermatan Sulfate in Normal and Inflamed Human Gingiva." *J. Dent. Res.* 71: 1587–93.

Becker, J., Schuppan, D. and Muller, S. 1993. "Immunohistochemical Distribution of Collagen Type I, 111, VI and VI, of Undulin and of Tenascin in Oral Fibrous Hyperplasia." *J. Oral Pathol. Med.* 22: 463–67.

Bhartiya, Deepa. 2013. "Are Mesenchymal Cells Indeed Pluripotent Stem Cells or Just Stromal Cells? OCT-4 and VSELs Biology Has Led to Better Understanding." *Stem Cells International* 2013. https://doi.org/10.1155/2013/547501.

Bhatavadekar, Neel B., and Amit S. Gharpure. 2018. "Controlled Palatal Harvest (CPH) Technique for Harvesting a Palatal Subepithelial Connective Tissue Graft." *Compend Clin Edu Dent* 39 (2).

Bosco, Alvaro Francisco. 2007. *An Alternative Technique to the Harvesting of a Connective Tissue Graft from a Thin Palate: Enhanced Wound Healing.*

Broome, William C., and Edward J. Taggart. 1976. "Free Autogenous Connective Tissue Grafting: Report of Two Cases." *Journal of Periodontology* 47 (10): 580–85. https://doi.org/10.1902/jop.1976.47.10.580.

Cazal, Cláudia, Ana Paula Veras Sobral, Ridel Frota Sá Nogueira Neves, Francisco Wagner Vasconcelos Freire Filho, Álvaro Bezerra Cardoso, and Márcia Maria Fonseca Da Silveira. 2008. "Oral Complaints in Progressive Systemic Sclerosis: Two Cases Report." *Medicina Oral, Patologia Oral y Cirugia Bucal* 13 (2): 114–18.

Chavrier, C. 1990. "The Elastic System Fibers in Healthy Human Gingiva." *Arch. Oral Biol.* 35: 223s-225s.

Chavrier, C., Couble, ML., Magloire, H. and Griniaud, JA. 1984. "Connective Tissue Organization of Healthy Human Gingiva. Ultrastructural Localization of Collagen Types." *J. Periodont Res.* 19: 221–29.

Culp, LA, Laterra J, Lark MW, Beyth RJ, Tobey SI.. 1986. "Heparan Sulphate Proteoglycan as Mediator of Some Adhesive Responses and

Cytoskeletal Reorganization of Cell and Iibroneain Matrices: Independent versus Cooperative Functions." *Ciba Found Symp* 124: 158–83.

John F. Bruno. *A Subepithelial Connective Tissue Graft Procedure for Optimum Root Coverage* September 1999 Vol 7, Issue 2, Pages 11–28.

de-Assis, Eliene Magda, Luiz Gustavo Garcia Santos Pimenta, Edson Costa-e-Silva, Paulo Eduardo Alencar Souza, and Martinho Campolina Rebello Horta. 2012. "Stromal Myofibroblasts in Oral Leukoplakia and Oral Squamous Cell Carcinoma." *Medicina Oral, Patologia Oral y Cirugia Bucal* 17 (5): 17–22. https://doi.org/10.4317/medoral.17834.

Del Pizzo, M., F Modica, N Bethaz, P Priotto, and Romagnoli R The. 2002. *The Connective Tissue Graft: A Comparative Clinical Evaluation of Wound Healing at the Palatal Donor Site*, 848–54.

Deliliers, GL, Santoro F, Polli N, Bohte E, Fumagalli L, and Risciotti E. 1986. "Light and Electronmicroscopic Study of Cyclosporin A-Induced Gingival Hyperplasia." *J Periodontol* 57: 771–77.

Deniz Çetiner,* Ay‚sen Bodur, and Ahu Uraz*, and Background: 2004. "Expanded Mesh Connective Tissue Graft for the Treatment Of." *J Periodontol* 75 (august): 1167–72.

Desmoulière, Alexis, Christelle Guyot, and Giulio Gabbiani. 2004. "The Stroma Reaction Myofibroblast: A Key Player in the Control of Tumor Cell Behavior." *International Journal of Developmental Biology* 48 (5–6): 509–17. https://doi.org/10.1387/ijdb.041802ad.

Dorfman, Albert. 1959. "The Biochemistry OF CONNECTIVE TISSUE." *J. Chron. Dis.* 10 (5): 403–17.

Edel. n.d. "Clinical Evaluation of Free Connective Tissue Grafts Used to Increase the Width of Keratinized Tissue. *Edel A. J Clin Periodontol* 1974;1-185-196.Pdf."

ElAttar, TMA, Hugoson, A. 1974. "Comparative Metabolism of Female Sex Steroids in Normal and Chronically Inflamed Gingiva of the Dog." *J Periodont Res* 9: 284–89.

Erlinger, R., Willerhausen-Zonnchen, B. and Welsch, U. 1995. "Ultrastructural Localization of Glycosaminoglycans in Human

Gingival Connective Tissue Using Cupromeronic Blue." *J. Periodont Res.* 30: 108-1 15.

Frank, CB., Shahla Khan, and Gulam S. Hashmi. 2004. "Histology and Functions of Connective Tissues." *University Journal of Dental Science* 4 (2): 1–2.

Fransson, LA. 1976. "Interaction between Dermatan Sulphate Chains. Affinity Chromatography of Copolymeric Galactosaminoglycans of Dermatan Sulphate Substituted Agarose." *Biochim Biophys Acra* 437: 106–15.

Gelse, K., E. Pöschl, and T. Aigner. 2003. "Collagens - Structure, Function, and Biosynthesis." *Advanced Drug Delivery Reviews* 55 (12): 1531–46. https://doi.org/10.1016/j.addr.2003.08.002.

Glickman I, Quintarelli J. 1960. "Further Observations Regarding the Effects of Ovariectomy upon the Tissues of the Periodontium." *J Periodontal.* 3 1: 3 1-7.

Gupta, MK, Shubhangi Mhaske, and Raju Ragavendra. 2008. "Oral Submucous Fibrosis -Current Concepts in Etiopathogenesis." *People's Journal of Scientific Research* 1 (July): 39–44.

Gupte, T, V Iyer, SG Damle, N Malik, and Halbe A Osteogenesis. 2017. *Osteogenesis Imperfecta* 24 (January): 6–9.

Harris, Randall J. 1994. "The Connective Tissue With Partial Thickness Double Pedicle Graft: The Results of 100 Consecutively-Treated Defects." *Journal of Periodontology* 65 (5): 448–61. https://doi.org/10.1902/jop.1994.65.5.448.

Hart, FD. n.d. "Anti-Inflammatory Drugs in the Treatment of Rheumatic Diseases." *Practitioner* 205: 597-603.

Hassan, Mohamed, Najma Latif, and Magdi Yacoub. 2012. "Adipose Tissue: Friend or Foe?" *Nature Reviews Cardiology* 9 (12): 689–702. https://doi.org/10.1038/nrcardio.2012.148.

Hassell, TM, Page RC, Narayaran AS, Cooper CG. 1976. "Diphenylhydantoin (Dilantin) Gingival Hyperplasia: Druginduced Abnormality of Connective Tissue." *Proc Natl Acad Sci (USA)* 73 (2): 909–12.

Hassell, TM. 1981. "Epilepsy and the Oral Manifestations of Phenytoin Therapy." *Basel: Karger.*

Hinz, Boris. 2007. "Formation and Function of the Myofibroblast during Tissue Repair." *Journal of Investigative Dermatology* 127 (3): 526–37. https://doi.org/10.1038/sj.jid.5700613.

Hurzeler, Markus B, and D D S Med. n.d. *A Single-Incision Tectinique to Harvest Subepittielial Connective Tissue Grafts from Ttie Paiate.*

Karthikeyan, BV., MLV. Prabhuji, Divya Khanna, and Kamedh Yashawant Chowdhary. 2016. "The Versatile Subepithelial Connective Tissue Graft: A Literature Update." *General Dentistry* 64 (6): e28–33.

Kashtan, Clifford. 2017. "Alport Syndrome: Facts and Opinions." *F1000Research* 6 (0): 2–9. https://doi.org/10.12688/f1000research.9636.1.

Kielty, Cay M., and Michael E. Grant. 2003. "The Collagen Family: Structure, Assembly, and Organization in the Extracellular Matrix." *Connective Tissue and Its Heritable Disorders*, 159–221. https://doi.org/10.1002/0471221929.ch2.

Kierszenbaum, AL, Abraham L. 2002. *Histology and Cell Biology—An Introduction to Pathology: St Louis (u.a): Mosby.*

Kofoed, JA, Houssay AB, Curbelo HM, Tocci AA, Gamper, and CH. 1973. "Effects of Glucocorticoids upon the Glycosaminoglycans in Salivary Glands in the Rat." *Arch Oral Biol* 18: 681–88.

Kornman, KS, Loesche WJ. 1980. "The Subgingival Microbial Flora during Pregnancy." *J Periodont Res* 15 (11): 1-2.

Kornman, KS, Loesche WJ 1982. *Effects of Estradiol and Progesterone on Bacreroides Melaninogenices and Bacteroides Gingivalis. Infection Immunity* 35: 256–63.

Kumar, Ashish, Vishal Sood, Sujata Surendra Masamatti, M. G. Triveni, D. S. Mehta, Manish Khatri, and Vipin Agarwal. 2013. "Modified Single Incision Technique to Harvest Subepithelial Connective Tissue Graft." *Journal of Indian Society of Periodontology* 17 (5): 676–80. https://doi.org/10.4103/0972-124X.119294.

Langer, Burton, and Lawrence Calagna. 1980. "The Subepithelial Connective Tissue Graft." *The Journal of Prosthetic Dentistry* 44 (4): 363–67. https://doi.org/10.1016/0022-3913(80)90090-6.

Larjava, H., HWinen, L. and Rahemtulla, F. 1992. "A Biochemical Analysis of Human Periodontal Tissue Proteoglycans." *Biochem. J.* 284: 261–74.

Larjava, H., Zhou, C., Larjava, 1. and Rahemtulla, F. 1992. "Immunolocalization of Beta 1 Integrins in Human Gingival Epithelium and Cultured Keratinocytes, Scand." *J. Dent. Res.* 100: 266–73.

Letourneau, Y, Perusse R, Buithieu H. 2001. "Oral Manifestations of Ehlers-Danlos Syndrome." *J Can Dent Assoc* 67: 330–34.

Light, Nicholas D, and Allen J Bailey. 1982. "Covalent Cross-Links in Collagen By." *Biochem. J.* 82: 360–72.

Lindhe, J, Branemark P-I, Lindskug J. 1967. "Changes in Vascular Proliferation after Local Application of Sex Hormones." *J Dent Res* 2: 266-72.

Lorenzana, Eduardo, and Edward P Allen. 2000. *The Single-Incision Palatal Harvest Technique: A Strategy for Esthetics and Patient Comfort*, no. February 2014.

Lourenço, Silvia V., Fabio R. G. De Carvalho, Paula Boggio, Mirian N. Sotto, Maria A. C. Vilela, Evandro A. Rivitti, and Marcello M. S. Nico. 2007. "Lupus Erythematosus: Clinical and Histopathological Study of Oral Manifestations and Immunohistochemical Profile of the Inflammatory Infiltrate." *Journal of Cutaneous Pathology* 34 (7): 558–64. https://doi.org/10.1111/j.1600-0560.2006.00652.x.

Maynes, R. 2012. *Structure and Function of Collagen Types.* Elsevier.

McLeod, Dwight E., and and Grishondra Branch-Mays Elio Reyes. 2009. "Case Report." *J Periodontol* 80 (10). https://doi.org/10.1902/jop.2009.090187.

Miller, EJ, Gay S. 1987. "The Collagens: An Overview and Update." *Methods in Enzymology* 144: 3-41.

Narayan, AS, Page RC. n.d. "Connective Tissues of the Periodontium: A Summary of Current Work. Collagen Rel Res ;3:33-64. 266 1991;36:4." *Australian Dental Journal*, 33–64.

Narayanan, AS. and Page, RC. n.d. "Connective Tissues of the Periodontiurn: A Summary of Current Work." *Collagen Re/. Rex* 3: 3 3 4 4.

Narayanan, AS. Page, RC. 1983. "Connective Tissues of the Periodontiurn: A Summary of Current Work, Collagen Re/. Rex."

Narayanan, AS., Clagett, JA. and Page, RC. 1985. "Effect of Inflammation on the Distribution of Collagen Types, I,III, IV, and V and Type I Trimer and Fibronectin in Human Gingivae." *J. Dent. Res.* 64: 1111-1116.

Nelson, SW. 1987. "The Subpedicle Connective Tissue Graft. A Bilaminar Reconstructive Procedure for the Coverage of Denuded Root Surfaces." *Journal of Periodontology* 58 (2): 95–102. https://doi.org/10.1902/jop.1987.58.2.95.

Neville, BW, Damm DD, Allen CM, Bouquot JE. 2009. *Oral and Maxillofacial Pathology (3rd Ed). St Louis: WB Saunders*.

Nimni, M. 1980. "The Molecular Organization of Collagen and Its Role in Determining the Biophysical Properties of the Connective Tissues." *Biorheology* 17: 51-82.

Nyman, S. 1971. "Studies of the Effect of Estradiol and Progesterone on Granulation Tissue." *J Periodont Res* Suppl 7: 1–24.

Parry, DA, Craig AS. 1984. "Growth and Development of Collagen Fibrils in Connective Tissue." In *Ultrastructure of the Connective Tissue Matrix*. In Springer, Boston, *MA.*, 34–36.

Pitaru, S., Aubin, JE., Bhargava, U. and Melcher, AH. 1987. "Immunoelectron Microscopic Studies on the Distributions of Fibronectin and Actin in a Cellular Dense Connective Tissue: The Periodontal Ligament of the Rat." *J. Periodont Res.* 22: 64–74.

Ponec, M. 1984. "Effects of Glucocorticoids on Cultured Skin Fibroblasts and Keratinocytes." *Int J Dermatol* 23: 11-24.

Ponle, AR, Rosenberg IC. 1987. "Proteoglycans, Chondrocalcin, and the Calcification of Cartilage Matrix in Endochondral Ossification." *Wight*

TN, Mecham RP, Eds. *Biology of Proteoglycans*. Orlando: Academic Press, 187-210.

Pontes, F, Rafael V Mantovani, Fernando S Ribeiro, Daniela L Zandim, and Ana Emı. 2008. *Case Report*, no. April: 753–58. https://doi.org/10.1902/jop.2008.070274.

Raetzke, Peter B. 1985. "Covering Localized Areas of Root Exposure Employing the 'Envelope' Technique." *Journal of Periodontology* 56 (7): 397–402. https://doi.org/10.1902/jop.1985.56.7.397.

Raines1, Matthew D. Shoulders1 and Ronald T. 2009. "COLLAGEN STRUCTURE AND STABILITY Matthew." *Annu Rev Biochem.* 78: 929–58. https://doi.org/10.1146/annurev.biochem.77.032207.120833. COLLAGEN.

Rainsford Marcel Dekker, KD. 1987. "Biochemical Effects of Anti-Inflammatory Drugs in Inflammatory Diseases." In: *Williamson WRN, Ed. Anti-Inflammatory Compounds*. New York.

Rajalalitha, P., and S. Vali. 2005. "Molecular Pathogenesis of Oral Submucous Fibrosis - A Collagen Metabolic Disorder." *Journal of Oral Pathology and Medicine* 34 (6): 321–28. https://doi.org/10.1111/j.1600-0714.2005.00325.x.

Ramakrishnan, T, Manmeet Kaur, and Kriti Aggarwal. 2011. *"Root Coverage Using Epithelial Embossed Connective Tissue Graft"* 22 (5): 726–28. https://doi.org/10.4103/0970-9290.93466.

Roman, A., A. Soancă, A. Kasaj, and S. I. Stratul. 2013. "Subepithelial Connective Tissue Graft with or without Enamel Matrix Derivative for the Treatment of Miller Class I and II Gingival Recessions: A Controlled Randomized Clinical Trial." *Journal of Periodontal Research* 48 (5): 563–72. https://doi.org/10.1111/jre.12039.

Romanos, G., Schrter-Kermani, C., Hinz, N. and Bemimoulin, J.-, and P. 1991. *Immunohistochemical Distribution of the Collagen Types IV, V, VI and Glycoprotein Laminin in the Healthy Rat, Marmoset (Callithrix Jacchus) and Human Gingivae*. 11: 125–32.

Romanos, GE., Schroter, KC., Hinz. N., Wachtel, HC. and, and JP. Bernimoulin. 1991. "Immunohistochemical Localization of Collagenous Components in Healthy Periodontal Tissues of the Rat and Marmoset (Callithrix Jaccus) 11. Distribution of Collagen Types IV, V and VI." *J. Periodont Res.* 26: 323-332.

Rose, Peter S., Nicholas U. Ahn, Howard P. Levy, Donna Magid, Joie Davis, Ruth M. Liberfarb, Paul D. Sponseller, and Clair A. Francomano. 2001. "The Hip in Stickler Syndrome." *Journal of Pediatric Orthopaedics* 21 (5): 657–63. https://doi.org/10.1097/00004694-200109000-00020.

Ross, R. 1975. "Connective Tissue Cells, Cell Proliferation and Synthesis of Extracellular Matrix-a Review." *Philosophical Transactions of the Royal Society of London. Series B, Biological Sciences* 271 (912): 247–59. https://doi.org/10.1098/rstb.1975.0049.

Rostock, MH, Fry HR, Turner JE. 1986. "Severe Gingival Overgrowth Associated with Cyclosporine Therapy." *J Periodontol* 57: 294–99.

Sandhu, Simarpreet Virk, Shruti Gupta, and Kartesh Singla. 2012. *Collagen in Health and Disease,* no. March. https://doi.org/10.5005/jp-journals-10026-1032.

Sasisekharan, V., and N. Yathindra. 1999. "The Madras Group and the Structure of Collagen." *Proceedings of the Indian Academy of Sciences: Chemical Sciences* 111 (1): 5–12. https://doi.org/10.1002/chin.199929302.

Sawada, T., Yamamoto, T., Yanagisawa, T., Takuma, S., and K. Hasegawa, H. and Watanabe. 1990. "Electron-Immunocytochemistry of Laminin and Type-IV Collagen in the Junctional Epithelium of Rat Molar Gingiva," *J. Periodonr Res.* 25: 372–76.

Scott, JE. 1988. "Proteoglycan-Fibriltar Collagen Interactions." *Biochem J* 252: 313–23.

Shibutani, T., Muruhashi, Y. and Iwayama, Y. 1989. "Immunohistochemical Localization of Chondroitin Sulfate and Dermatan Sulfate Proteoglycan in Human Gingival Connective Tissue." *J. Periodont. Res.,* 24: 3 1 0-3 13.

Shukla, Anjani Kumar, Ravi Kumar, and Ashok Kumar. 2017. *"Correlation of Clinical Grading to Various Chewing Habits Factors with Oral Submucous Fibrosis: A Cross Sectional Study"* 3 (9): 23–25.

Silva, Elaine Zayas Marcelino da, Maria Célia Jamur, and Constance Oliver. 2014. *Mast Cell Function: A New Vision of an Old Cell. Journal of Histochemistry and Cytochemistry.* Vol. 62. https://doi.org/10.1369/0022155414545334.

Southern, AL, Rapport SC, Gordon GG. 1978. "Specific 5a Dihydrotestosterone Receptors in Human Gingiva." *J Clin Endocrinol Metab* 47: 1378–82.

Steffensen, B., Duong, AH., Milam, SB., Potempa, CL., and RJ. Winborn, WB., Magnuson, VL., Chen, D., Zardeneta, G. Klebe. n.d. "Immunohistological Localization of Cell Adhesion Proteins and Integrins in the Periodontium, " *J. Periodontol.,* 63: 584–92.

Stimmelmayr, M, Allen EP, Reichert TE, Iglhaut G. 2010. "Use of a Combination Epithelized-Subepithelial Connective Tissue Graft for Closure and Soft Tissue Augmentation of an Extraction Site Following Ridge Preservation or Implant Placement: Description of a Technique." *International Journal of Periodontics & Restorative Dentistry.* 1 (30): 4.

Tilakaratne, WM., MF. Klinikowski, Takashi Saku, TJ. Peters, and Saman Warnakulasuriya. 2006. "Oral Submucous Fibrosis: Review on Aetiology and Pathogenesis." *Oral Oncology* 42 (6): 561–68. https://doi.org/10.1016/j.oraloncology.2005.08.005.

Touyz, LZG.1984. "Vitamin C, Oral Scurvy and Periodontal Disease." *SA Med J* 65: 838–42.

Troyer, Deryl L., and Mark L. Weiss. 2008. "Concise Review: Wharton's Jelly-Derived Cells Are a Primitive Stromal Cell Population." *Stem Cells* 26 (3): 591–99. https://doi.org/10.1634/stemcells.2007-0439.

Ushiki, Tatsuo. 2002. "Collagen Fibers, Reticular Fibers and Elastic Fibers. A Comprehensive Understanding from a Morphological Viewpoint." *Archives of Histology and Cytology.* https://doi.org/10.1679/aohc.65.109.

Vittek, J, Hernandez MR, Wenk EJ, Rappapon SC, Southern, and AL. 1982. "Specific Estrogen Receptors in Human Gingiva." *J Clin Endocrinol Metab* 54: 608–12.

Vittek, J, Rapport SC, Gordon GC, Munangi PR, Southern, and AL. 1979. "Concentration of Circulating Hormones and Metabolism of Androgens by Human Gingiva." *J Periodontal.* 254–64.

Vuorio, E. 1990. "The Family of Collagen Genes." *Annual Review of Biochemistry* 59 (1): 837–72. https://doi.org/10.1146/annurev.biochem.59.1.837.

Wever, Olivier De, Pieter Demetter, Marc Mareel, and Marc Bracke. 2008. "Stromal Myofibroblasts Are Drivers of Invasive Cancer Growth." *International Journal of Cancer* 123 (10): 2229–38. https://doi.org/10.1002/ijc.23925.

Wheater's., Young B. Health JW. n.d. *Functional Histology: A Text and Colour Atlas 4th Edition.*

Williams, RC, Jeffcoat MK, Kaplan ML, et al. 1985. "Flubiprofen: A Potent Inhibitor of Alveolar Bone Resorption in Beagles." *Science.* 227: 640–42.

Yen, Jui Lung, Shuan Pei Lin, Ming Ren Chen, and Dau Ming Niu. 2006. "Clinical Features of Ehlers-Danlos Syndrome." *Journal of the Formosan Medical Association* 105 (6): 475–80. https://doi.org/10.1016/S0929-6646(09)60187-X.

Yeo, JF., 1986. "Binucleated Form of Plasma Cells in Oral Lesions--Their 'Vital Statistics'." *Ann Acad Med Singapore.* 15 (3): 365–69.

Zucchelli, Giovanni, Monica Mele, Martina Stefanini, Claudio Mazzotti, Matteo Marzadori, Lucio Montebugnoli, and Massimo De Sanctis. 2010. "Patient Morbidity and Root Coverage Outcome after Subepithelial Connective Tissue and De-Epithelialized Grafts: A Comparative Randomized-Controlled Clinical Trial." *Journal of Clinical Periodontology* 37 (8): 728–38. https://doi.org/10.1111/j.1600-051X.2010.01550.x.

In: Connective Tissue
Editor: Jim M. Pearson

ISBN: 978-1-53617-875-3
© 2020 Nova Science Publishers, Inc.

Chapter 2

CONNECTIVE TISSUE GRAFT

Shruti Bhatnagar

Department of Periodontology, Rungta College of Dental Sciences and Research (Pt. D.D.U Memorial and Ayush Uni. of C.G), Bhilai-Durg, Chhattisgarh, India

ABSTRACT

Connective tissue graft is a promising and reliable method that provides a satisfactory esthetic outcome, making it a popular alternative for clinicians. It can be described as a free autogenous graft. The surgical procedure was first described by Alan Edel in 1974 for increase in width of attached gingiva. It is generally used to obtain root coverage following gingival recession, which was a later development by Burt Langer in the early 1980s. The SCTG is obtained usually from the palatal area, tuberosity area, retromolar pad area too. The advantages of the SCTG are that it is inexpensive, versatile, and easily available; it provides successful outcomes; it is less invasive than other autogenous harvesting techniques; and it has a shorter healing period. Apart from this SCTG also have osteogenic, chondrogenic and mesenchymal properties. A connective tissue graft also could be used as a barrier for furcation defects and intrabony defects.

Keywords: subepithelial connective tissue graft, gingival recession, periodontal plastic surgery, healing

INTRODUCTION

Connective tissue graft or subepithelial connective tissue graft (SCTG) refers to the autogenous soft tissue procured from the palatal masticatory mucosa. The SCTG is devoid of overlying epithelium but the underneath connective tissue. It is widely used in periodontal plastic procedures such as root coverage, ridge augmentation, increasing width of attached gingiva and peri-implant plastic surgeries. [1] Recently some studies have shown use of it as guided tissue regeneration. [2]

SCTG was preceded by free gingival grafts in various periodontal plastic surgeries; however the desirous characteristics of SCTG such as reliable and predictable procedure providing a satisfactory esthetic outcome made it a popular alternative for clinicians. Major advantages of the SCTG are that it is inexpensive, versatile, and easily available; it provides successful outcomes; it is less invasive than other autogenous harvesting techniques; and it has a shorter healing period. [3-5]

The Cochrane review in 2010 has shown that gain in keratinized tissue and root coverage is better when compared with other modalities for the similar procedures. [6] The finding in the review were in accordance with findings of the analysis by Chambrone and Tatakis in their systematic review confirming that greater percentage of root coverage and keratinized tissue was obtained by SCTG. [7]

HISTORICAL BACKGROUND

Langer and Calagna in 1980 introduced a SCTG for soft tissue augmentation. [8] Langer & Langer (1985) introduced a palatal flap approach that allowed for harvesting of SCTG for treatment of gingival recession. [9] Their technique eliminated many unwanted results associated with free gingival graft technique which includes both quantitative and qualitative outcomes such as insufficient augmentation in terms of volume, poor esthetic integration, surface texture, and colour, scarring. [10] Nelson (1987) modified the procedure somewhat to further enhance clinical predictability (≥90%). [11]

The method of obtaining the tissue from palatal mucosa has been updated from time to time. Edel in 1974 introduced a trap door approach for procuring SCTG. He advocated use of oral mucosa rich in subepithelial tissue such as from palatal mucosa, maxillary tuberosity or edentulous area. Raetzke (1985) used two converging horizontal incisions. Harris (1992) used a specialized knife with two blade marking two horizontal incisions. Hurzeler et al., 1999; Lorenzana et al., 2000 used an envelope technique. Del Pizzo et al. 2002 advised a single incision technique. Ribeiro et al. used a split CTG technique. Kumar et al. used a Modified Hurzeler and Weng single incision technique. [2, 5]

SURGICAL CONSIDERATIONS

The harvesting of donor tissue from the subepithelial connective tissue of the palate requires thorough knowledge of the entire palate. The palate consists of masticatory mucosa consisting of orthokeratinized epithelial layer and a thick, even stratum corneum, compared with gingiva that has an inhomogeneous stratum corneum of varying thickness and an orthokeratinized or parakeratinized surface. The epithelium of both hard palate and gingiva have an average thickness of 0.3 mm [12] and a maximum thickness of 0.6 mm. [13] The lamina propria or connective tissue of the palate extends to a depth of approximately 1.25 to 3.0 mm, and then submucosa extends from there to the bone. [8]

The palatal soft tissue which extends superiorly from the CEJ of the maxillary posterior teeth (for approximately 2 to 3 mm) and the soft tissue near the median palatal raphe are composed of very dense lamina propria, which is directly bound to periosteum. The masticatory mucosa between these two sites is the common location of the donor sites for most connective tissue grafts and is composed of connective tissue and loosely organized glandular and adipose tissue. [13] The pars corporis adiposa contains adipose tissue and resides in the area of the premolars, whereas the pars corporis glandulosum contains glandular tissue and extends posteriorly to the soft palate [14]; the two are roughly separated by the thin mucosa over the palatal root of the first molar. [15] When the density of connective tissue decreases and becomes loosely organized, the thickness of the donor tissue must be increased or it will be too thin to manipulate and will tear while trying to suture the graft. The best quality connective tissue is found closest to the teeth rather than the midline of the palate; however, taking tissue closer than 2 mm to the teeth puts those teeth at risk for postoperative gingival recession. If the donor connective tissue is taken too close to the epithelial layer, the retained flap will not have an adequate blood supply and the palatal flap will slough giving a similar type wound as an epithelialized donor graft wound. [8]

Another important consideration during harvesting is position of the greater and lesser palatine arteries and nerves in the surgical field. Clinician must be well aware of their location. The greater and lesser palatine foramens are located apical to the third molar at the junction of the vertical and horizontal components of the palate. The greater and lesser palatine vessels and nerves lie in a bony groove, the greater palatine groove, which traverses the palate anteriorly at the junction of the horizontal and vertical palate. The nerves and vessels located along this neurovascular line should be avoided. The location of this line varies relative to the CEJ—in shallow palatal vaults the minimal distance is 7 mm, whereas in high vaults the maximum distance can be up to 17 mm. In an average vault there is a distance of 12 mm from the neurovascular line to the CEJ. [13] If the incision is started 2 mm from the soft tissue margin and is ended 2 mm from the neurovascular line, then the maximum width of donor tissue will vary from 3 mm in the shallow vault to 13 mm in the high vault, with an average width of 8 mm in the average vault. The width of connective tissue needed for most grafts is determined by the extent of root exposure and the amount of root coverage anticipated, but 5 to 9 mm is usually an adequate width for donor tissue. This means removing a connective tissue graft from an individual with a shallow palate may result in trauma to the neurovascular structures; thus only 3 to 5 mm of donor tissue can be taken before risking damage to a vessel or nerve.

When connective tissue is taken for ridge augmentation, the maximum amount of soft tissue is often desired, and the amount of tissue available is relative to the anatomy as described earlier. These limitations in length, width, and thickness are the reasons other sources of donor connective tissues are being evaluated. [8]

INDICATIONS

The use of SCTG varies from soft tissue augmentation to root coverage and improving aesthetic outcomes around implants. Use of SCTG for increasing width of attached gingiva has also given promising results. Papilla reconstruction and augmentation is another use of SCTG. It can be used as a barrier membrane too in intra osseous defects. SCTG can also be used for correction of gingival pigmentation. [5]

ADVANTAGES

Dual blood supply, carries a genetic message, better colour matching, improved aesthetic outcome, greater predictability, primary healing and less discomfort at donor site, autogenous and cost effective

DISADVANTAGES

Extra surgical site, requires precision, technique sensitive, may require special armamentarium (only in certain techniques)

Techniques for Harvesting SCTG

The methods of harvesting SCTG vary considerably. The techniques from single incision technique as initially proposed by Edel to double incision techniques. Vertical incisions are also employed. The following is the description of various technique developed over the years.

Edel (1974) [16] has given trapdoor technique. The technique consists of primary incision is made along the long axis of the teeth, near the gingival margin. A total of 1 horizontal and 2 vertical incisions are made, the flap is raised, and the graft is harvested. The under surface of an edentulous region can also be used for harvesting the graft. Complete wound closure is achieved, hence primary healing is achieved. However vertical incisions may compromise blood supply. [1, 5]

Langer & Calagna (1980) [17] proposed a horizontal bevel incision on the palate 1 mm apical to the free gingival margin of the teeth. This is followed by vertical incisions at either end, and the graft is harvested from the palatal side. The graft is obtained along with a band of epithelium. This leads to better merging of epithelial junction at the recipient site and decreased graft shrinkage. But vertical incision may pose a problem at donor site. [1, 5]

Langer & Langer (1985) [9] have given a rectangular design, with 2 horizontal and 2 vertical incisions resulting in an SCTG with an epithelial collar of 1.5-2.0 mm in width. They followed the previous method of having a layer of epithelium and explained dual blood supply. Healing is by secondary intention due to incomplete closure at the donor site. [1, 5]

Raetzke (1985) [18] proposed 2 converging horizontal, crescent-shaped incisions that intersect deep within the palate, sparing bone, producing a wedge of SCTG with an epithelial collar. No vertical incisions are given. Healing is by primary intention. The graft obtained is limited and hence not suitable for multiple recessions. It epithelium is removed in the procedure healing would occur by secondary intention. [1, 5]

Harris (1992) [19] has given a double blade technique, a modification of original trapdoor technique; a graft knife is used to elevate a split-thickness flap, which is attached to the palate distally. The knife is then pulled mesially under the trapdoor flap, starting at the distal edge of the connective tissue, to elevate an SCTG. The technique can be simplified by utilizing a Harris double-bladed graft knife, an instrument with two blades mounted 1.5 mm apart. The use of double blade provides a graft of uniform thickness. However epithelium is also removed along with underlying connective tissue, resulting into incomplete closure of wound. [1, 5]

Hürzeler & Weng (1999) [20] proposed a single horizontal incision technique. Incision is made on the palate, 2 mm away from marginal gingiva. At first blade is angled to 90 degrees, after then it is angled to 135 degrees to undermine the flap. The SCTG is removed by making the incision to the bone on all sides of the uncovered SCTG. Advantages of using this technique are: Sloughing of epithelium due to an unfavourable relationship between the flap base and pedicle length will be avoided, postoperative healing is better, and patient morbidity is decreased. [10] The lack of vertical incision may pose a problem in access. [1, 5]

Bruno (1994) [21] put forward a double incision technique in which first incision is made perpendicular to the long axis of the teeth about 2-3 mm apical to the gingival margin of the maxillary teeth, avoiding bone closely. The second incision is made parallel to the long axis of the teeth but 1-2 mm apical to the first incision. A small periosteal elevator is used to raise a full-thickness periosteal SCTG along with overlying epithelium. No vertical incisions are given. [1, 5]

Lorenzana & Allen (2000) [22] technique is similar to as the one described by Hürzeler & Weng, but vertical (mesial and distal) and medial incisions are not made to relieve the graft. Careful manipulation of the graft with tissue forceps is required to avoid compression or tearing of the graft. Healing occurs by primary intention with procurement of adequate quantity of graft. Proper visibility may be a problem due to no vertical incision. [1, 5]

Del Pizzo et al. (2002) [23] single incision for access is extended up to the bone perpendicular to the palatal tissue surface. Through this incision, a split-thickness dissection is made parallel to the long axis of the teeth to dissect the graft from underlying bone and superficial tissues. No blunt dissection with periosteal elevator is made, leaving the periosteum on the bone surface, thus ensuring blood supply at donor site. This approach aids in the formation of granulation tissue at the wound and hastens the repair of the palatal donor site. The procedure requires precision. [1, 5]

Bosco & Bosco (2007) [24] advised split-thickness flap to be raised from the edges of a 1.5-mm incision, keeping the periosteum intact. A thick graft, consisting of the epithelium and connective tissue, is harvested. The graft is placed on a sterile cloth and bisected. One of the resulting grafts consists of epithelium with connective tissue, while the other consists only of connective tissue. The epithelial graft is repositioned at the donor site like a free gingival graft and periodontal dressing is placed, with or without compression sutures. This technique helps in obtaining the graft even from shallow palatal vault. The graft obtained is usually contains less amount of adipose or glandular tissue. Bisecting of graft however may result in graft perforation at times resulting in compromise in blood supply. [1, 5]

Ribeiro et al. (2008) [25] proposed single-incision technique used to harvest the SCTG with maximum thickness so that it can be split cross-sectionally. However, the graft is not divided completely into 2 parts; therefore, it is almost double the length of the original graft and has a thickness of approximately 1.5 mm. Thus quantity of graft is not an issue in this technique. The procedure is not consistent in case of thin mucosa on palate. Obtaining uniform thickness may also be a problem. [1, 5]

McLeod et al. (2009) [26] described sharp back-action periodontal surgical chisel is used to de-epithelialize the palatal donor site from the mesial aspect of the canine to the distal aspect of the first molar. After de-epithelialization, the SCTG is harvested with a surgical blade in the manner used to harvest a conventional free gingival graft. A uniform and adequate graft is obtained through this procedure. No sutures are required. Technique will provide enough graft for multiple recessions. Care should be taken to avoid vasculature as de-epithelisation approaches midline. [1]

Kumar et al. (2103) [27] modified Hurzeler and Weng single incision technique in which first incision is of partial thickness. Less bleeding; better visibility, better estimation of the connective tissue graft size, and better control over the incisions, as there are no arbitrary angulations to be followed are advantages of this technique; new AVS instrument and Barraquer cataract knife are useful to overcome the difficulties faced by operators in making medial and vertical incisions respectively; it requires reduced number of sutures compared to conventional techniques. [1]

Bhatavadekar and Gharpure (2018) [28] proposed a controlled palatal harvest technique. It involves obtaining the graft from inner surface of full thickness flap. It provides adequate control due to good visibility, good predictability in ensuring adequate graft and flap thickness, ability to obtain uniform graft and flap thickness, and less chance of leaving behind a thin flap for closure at the donor site thereby minimizing necrosis and flap sloughing and improving grafting success. Disadvantages include technique-sensitivity and dependence on the thickness of the palatal mucosa. In cases with thin mucosa, there is a chance of perforation of the flap while obtaining the graft; harvest procedure is done from a relatively mobile flap; greater clinician skill is required compared to conventional techniques; as with any incision perpendicular to the blood supply, increased bleeding is possible. [1]

CLINICAL CONSIDERATIONS

The various procedures done using SCTG are root coverage, ridge augmentation, mucogingval surgeries around implants and SCTG as barrier membrane.

Root Coverage [11]

The procedure is basically a combination of a partial-thickness coronally positioned flap and a free connective tissue graft.

Recipient Site: (1) The root surface is scaled and root planed to flatten prominent convexities and to remove any softened root structure, endotoxins, and composite restorations. Enamel finishing burs may be used to help flatten the root convexity in the central portion of the root or after removal of composite restorations. (2) Use of the chemical root modifiers citric acid (pH 1.0 for 3 to 5 minutes) tetracycline (3 to 5 minutes) or ethylene diamine tetra acetic acid (EDTA) (pH 7.0) is optional. (3) A no. 15 scalpel is used to outline the surgical site, making sure to raise a partial-thickness flap (no incisions are made down to bone). The scalloped papillary incisions must be made above the CEJ to assume total root coverage and so that an adequate bleeding surface is prepared. (4) Two vertical incisions are extended adequately into the mucosal tissues to permit coronal positioning of the flap. The partial thickness flap is raised by sharp dissection. (5) Apically, the undersurface of the flap is released from the underlying periosteum via a horizontal incision. This will permit coronal positioning of the flap. [11]

Donor Site: (1) A straight, horizontal incision is begun approximately 5 to 6 mm from the free gingival margin with a no. 15 scalpel blade. The incision is begun in the molar areas and extended anteriorly. The blade is used to undermine a partial-thickness palatal flap. (2) A second, more coronally positioned parallel incision is now made approximately 3 mm from the gingival margin with a no. 15 blade. It is continued apically to the same level as the first incision. The blade may have to be angled toward the bone to ensure adequate graft thickness. (3) Vertical incisions (optional) are used for graft release mesially and distally. They are made from the outer epithelial surface down through the submucosa. This will free the terminal ends of the graft. (4) To completely free the graft, a horizontal incision is made at its most apical border. (5) On removal, the graft is placed on a saline moistened gauze sponge. (6) The palate is now sutured with a combination of horizontal mattress sutures or continuous sutures. Immediate suturing will promote hemostasis and prevent excessive clot formation. [11]

Graft Placement: (1) The graft is trimmed to size with a sharp scissors or no. 15 blade. There is no need for complete removal of glandular or fatty tissue. (2) The graft is placed so that the epithelial border is positioned above the CEJ and onto the enamel. This will ensure greater root coverage, predictability, and enhanced aesthetics. (3) Intimate graft-root contact is achieved by first stabilizing the graft laterally with interrupted sutures and then by using a continuous sling suture about the necks of the teeth for cervical positioning and stabilization. To avoid problems of retrieval, chromic gut sutures are recommended for graft positioning and stabilization. 4. The primary flap is now coronally positioned and sutured with 4-0 silk (P-3 needle) to cover as much of the graft as possible. The flap is positioned laterally with interrupted sutures and coronally with a suspensory sling suture. [11]

The graft can be completely covered at the recipient site or may remain partially covered.

Partially Covered Connective Tissue Graft

The partially covered connective tissue graft was originally described by Langer and Langer. [9] The technique can be used for Class I, II, or III recession defects. The grafted connective tissue when partially covered, the blood supply was not as good as if the donor tissue was completely covered by a coronally positioned facial flap. The donor tissue must be thick enough to survive over the avascular root of the tooth, and in this case the tissue was a thick graft (1.5 to 2.0 mm thick). The grafted tissue may not look as normal as with the completely covered connective tissue graft; however, the colour match can be very close. Once healing is complete, minor gingivoplasty is sometimes needed to blend the tissue at each papilla. The advantage of this partial graft coverage technique is that the mucogingival junction and the vestibular depth maintain their preoperative dimensions, whereas with a completely covered connective tissue graft, the vestibule becomes more shallow and the mucogingival junction moves incisally because of the coronal positioning of the flap. Also is that when the connective tissue is exposed, it keratinizes and increases the width of keratinized gingiva. [29] The major disadvantage is that thick donor tissue may not always be available, and thinner tissue requires more coverage with the overlying flap. [8]

Completely Covered Connective Tissue Graft

The completely covered connective tissue graft uses a coronally positioned flap either with vertical incisions or with horizontal incisions. The decision to use vertical incisions is the same as with the coronally positioned flap; vertical incisions allow more flap advancement but decreased blood supply and slight scarring of the mucosa. In most cases, the horizontal technique is used initially because vertical incisions can be made if necessary to increase the coronal advancement of the flap. This technique is indicated for Class I recession defects when a thin or average connective tissue graft can be placed under the coronally positioned flap to thicken the soft tissue complex. In Class I defects, a band of keratinized tissue is present at the recipient site before grafting. [8] The advantages of completely covering a connective tissue graft include better aesthetics and the ability to use a thinner graft. A thin graft may not survive over a root surface if it is not completely covered; therefore, a thin connective tissue graft is generally covered completely with a pedicle flap. When a thin connective tissue graft (0.5 to 0.8 mm) is placed under a thin flap (0.5 to 0.8), the total thickness is 1 to 1.6 mm, which closely mimics the thickness of normal gingiva. [30] An average thickness graft is often completely covered by an advanced flap, but it is not mandatory. The goal is to have marginal gingiva that is at least 1 mm in thickness. If small areas of the graft are exposed, they will often survive, especially if the collagen content is high and tissue quality is good. [8]

Ridge Augmentation

Ridge augmentation using connective tissue grafts was first described by Langer and Calagna in 1980. If the overlying facial tissue is thick, a split-thickness flap is dissected leaving a connective tissue bed. If the gingiva is thin, a full-thickness flap is reflected with a deep periosteal releasing incision making the base of the flap a split-thickness flap with mobility to advance the flap. The connective tissue donor tissue is taken from the palate, and it should be thicker than is needed if possible. The donor tissue is secured with 6–0 absorbable sutures until it is immobile. It is easier to secure the donor tissue if a split-thickness flap is reflected because the connective tissue bed allows better stabilization. If a full-thickness flap is used, the donor tissue must be sutured to the wound edges and with horizontal stabilizing sutures through the facial flap when necessary. [8]

SCTG for Implant Esthetics

The peri-implant aesthetics can also be maintained using subepithelial connective tissue graft. The harvested tissue can be placed around implant fixtures by raising mucoperiosteal flap. [31, 32]

SCTG as Barrier Membrane

A subepithelial connective tissue graft (SCTG) also could be used as a barrier for furcation defects and infrabony defects. Palatal connective tissue graft is autogenous membranes which have shown successful results in the previous studies. [33] Mesenchymal cells are seen in the palatal connective tissue, and these cells are osteogenic. [34] It was proposed that the gingival connective tissue contains mesenchymal cells. These cells are osteogenic, chondrogenic, osteoblastic, and have immunomodulatory capacity. [35]

HEALING

The success of the graft depends on survival of the connective tissue. Sloughing of the epithelium occurs in most cases, but the extent to which the connective tissue withstands the transfer to the new location determines the fate of the graft. Fibrous organization of the interface between the graft and the recipient bed occurs within 2 to several days. [36, 37]

The graft is initially maintained by a diffusion of fluid from the host bed, adjacent gingiva, and alveolar mucosa. [38] The fluid is a transudate from the host vessels and provides nutrition and hydration essential for the initial survival of the transplanted tissues. During the first day, the connective tissue becomes edematous and disorganized and undergoes degeneration and lysis of some of its elements. As healing progresses, the edema is resolved, and degenerated connective tissue is replaced by new granulation tissue. [36]

Revascularization of the graft starts by the second or third day. Capillaries from the recipient bed proliferate into the graft to form a network of new capillaries and anastomose with preexisting vessels. [39]

Many of the graft vessels degenerate and are replaced by new ones, and some participate in the new circulation. The central section of the surface is the last to vascularize, but this is complete by the tenth day. [36]

The epithelium undergoes degeneration and sloughing, with complete necrosis occurring in some areas. [40, 41] It is replaced by new epithelium from the borders of the recipient site. A thin layer of new epithelium is present by the fourth day, with rete pegs developing by the seventh day. [36]

As seen microscopically, healing of a graft of intermediate thickness (0.75 mm) is complete by 10.5 weeks; thicker grafts (1.75 mm) may require 16 weeks or longer. [42] The gross appearance of the graft reflects the tissue changes within it. At transplantation the graft vessels are empty and the graft is pale. The pallor changes to an ischemic grayish white during the first 2 days until vascularization begins and a pink color appears. The plasmatic circulation accumulates and causes softening and swelling of the graft, which are reduced when the edema is removed from the recipient site by the new blood vessels. Loss of epithelium leaves the graft smooth and shiny. New epithelium creates a thin, gray, veil-like surface that develops normal features as the epithelium matures. [36]

Functional integration of the graft occurs by the seventeenth day, but the graft is morphologically distinguishable from the surrounding tissue for months. The graft eventually blends with adjacent tissues, but sometimes, although pink, firm, and healthy, it is somewhat bulbous. This usually presents no problem, but if the graft traps plaque or is esthetically unacceptable, thinning of the graft may be necessary. Thinning the surface of the grafted tissue does reduce the bulbous condition because the surface epithelium tends to proliferate again. The graft should be thinned by making the necessary incisions to elevate it from the periosteum, removing tissue from its undersurface, and suturing it back in place. [36]

COMPLICATIONS

Donor site complications [43]: necrosis of graft and palatal site, pain and excessive haemorrhage, protracted discomfort, increased chances of infection at donor site, in rare cases, loss of sensation in palate.

Recipient site complications [5]: Postsurgical swelling and ecchymosis, external root resorption, gingival cysts, gingival soft tissue abscess, exostosis, graft loss, epithelial cell discharge, reaction to suture material, gingival cul-de-sac defects, suturing under tension, thereby impinging on microcirculation

Causes of subepithelial connective tissue graft failure or failure to provide root coverage [44]:

- Insufficient height of interdental bone
- Reflection of all interdental papilla
- Horizontal incision placed apical to cementoenamel junction
- Flap penetration
- Graft that is too thick or too thin
- Tension in graft
- Ineffective postsurgical biofilm control during healing
- Inadequate height and thickness of keratinized tissue

CONCLUSION

SCTG has been the gold standard when it comes to root coverage. The predictable outcomes and efficiency has contributed to its popularity in periodontal plastic surgery. The new scope of SCTG in implant aesthetics and barrier membrane broadens the spectrum of its use. The variations in harvesting techniques of the graft over the period of time only define its effectiveness in the field. The clinicians have to be adept with the advancement as well as the methods of SCTG to keep up with the same.

REFERENCES

[1] Puri K., Kumar A., Khatri M., Bansal M., Rehan M., Siddeshappa S. T. (2019). 44-year journey of palatal connective tissue graft harvest: A narrative review. *Journal of Indian Society of Periodontology*, 23(5): 395-408.

[2] Siddeshappa S. T., Bhatnagar S., Diwan V., Parvez H. (2018). Regenerative potential of subepithelial connective tissue graft in the treatment of periodontal infrabony defects. *Journal of Indian Society of Periodontology*, 22(6): 492-497.

[3] Harris R. J. (1999). Successful root coverage: a human histologic evaluation of a case. *International Journal of Periodontics and Restorative Dentistry*, 19(5): 439-447.

[4] Zuhr O., Bäumer D., Hürzeler M. (2014). The addition of soft tissue replacement grafts in plastic periodontal and implant surgery: critical elements in design and execution. *Journal of Clinical Periodontology*, 41(Suppl 15): S123-S142.

[5] Karthikeyan B. V., Khanna D., Chowdhary K. Y., Prabhuji M. L. (2016). The versatile subepithelial connective tissue graft: a literature update. *General Dentistry*, 64(6): e28-e33.

[6] Chambrone L., Sukekava F., Araújo M. G., *et al.* (2010). Root-coverage procedures for the treatment of localized

recession-type defects: A Cochrane systematic review. *Journal of Periodontology,* 81(4): 452-478.

[7] Chambrone L., Tatakis D. N. (2015). Periodontal soft tissue root coverage procedures: A systematic review from the AAP regeneration workshop. *Journal of Periodontology,* 86(2 Suppl): S8-51.

[8] Rose Louis F., Mealey Brian, Genco Robert, Cohen D. Walter. *Periodontics: Medicine, Surgery and Implants,* (Elsevier Mosby, Philadelphia, 2004).

[9] Langer B., Langer L. (1985). Subepithelial connective tissue graft technique for root coverage. *Journal of Periodontology*, 56(12): 715-720.

[10] Zuhr O., Bäumer D., Hürzeler M. (2014). The addition of soft tissue replacement grafts in plastic periodontal and implant surgery: critical elements in design and execution. *Journal of Clinical Periodontology,* 41(Suppl 15): S123-S142.

[11] Cohen Edward S. (*Atlas of Cosmetic and Reconstructive Periodontal Surgery*, PMPH – USA, 2007).

[12] Schroeder H. *Differentiation of human oral stratified epithelia,* (Basel, Switzerland, 1981), Karger AG.

[13] Reiser G., Bruno J., Mahan P. E., Larkin L. H. (1996). The subepithelial connective tissue graft palatal donor site: anatomic considerations for surgeons. *International Journal of Periodontics and Restorative Dentistry*, 16(2): 131–137.

[14] Schroeder H. *Oral structural biology,* New York, 1991, Thieme, 350–370.

[15] Muller H., Eger T. (2002). Masticatory mucosa and periodontal phenotype: a review, *International Journal of Periodontics and Restorative Dentistry*, 22(2): 172–183.

[16] Edel A. (1974). Clinical evaluation of free connective tissue grafts used to increase the width of keratinised gingiva. *Journal of Clinical Periodontology,* 1(4): 185-196.

[17] Langer B., Calagna L. (1980). The subepithelial connective tissue graft. *Journal of Prosthetic Dentistry,* 44(4): 363-367.

[18] Raetzke P. B. (1985). Covering localized areas of root exposure employing the "envelope" technique. *Journal of Periodontology*, 56(7): 397-402.

[19] Harris R. J. (1992). The connective tissue and partial thickness double pedicle graft: a predictable method of obtaining root coverage. *Journal of Periodontology*, 63(5): 477-486.

[20] Hürzeler M. B., Weng D. (1999). A single-incision technique to harvest subepithelial connective tissue grafts from the palate. *International Journal of Periodontics and Restorative Dentistry*, 19(3): 279-287.

[21] Bruno J. F. (1994). Connective tissue graft technique assuring wide root coverage. *International Journal of Periodontics and Restorative Dentistry*, 14(2): 126-137.

[22] Lorenzana E. R., Allen E. P. (2000). The single-incision palatal harvest technique: A strategy for esthetics and patient comfort. *International Journal of Periodontics and Restorative Dentistry*, 20(3):297-305.

[23] Del Pizzo M., Modica F., Bethaz N., Priotto P., Romagnoli R. (2002). The connective tissue graft: a comparative clinical evaluation of wound healing at the palatal donor site. A preliminary study. *Journal of Clinical Periodontology,* 29(9): 848-854.

[24] Bosco A. F., Bosco J. M. (2007). An alternative technique to the harvesting of a connective tissue graft from a thin palate: enhanced wound healing. *International Journal of Periodontics and Restorative Dentistry*, 27(2): 133-139.

[25] Ribeiro F. S., Zandim D. L., Pontes A. E., Mantovani R. V., Sampaio J. E., Marcantonio E. (2008). Tunnel technique with a surgical maneuver to increase the graft extension: case report with a 3-year follow- up. *Journal of Periodontology*, 79(4): 753-758.

[26] McLeod D. E., Reyes E., Branch-Mays G. (2009). Treatment of multiple areas of gingival recession using a simple harvesting technique for autogenous connective tissue graft. *Journal of Periodontology*, 80(10): 1680-1687.

[27] Kumar A., Sood V., Masamatti S. S., et al. (2013). Modified single incision technique to harvest subepithelial connective tissue graft. *Journal of Indian Society of Periodontology,* 17(5): 676-80.

[28] Bhatavadekar N. B., Gharpure A. S. (2018). Controlled palatal harvest technique for harvesting a palatal subepithelial connective tissue graft. *Compendium of Continuing Education in Dentistry,* 39(2): e9-e12.

[29] Cordiolo G., Mortarino C., Chierico A., et al. (2001). Comparison of 2 techniques of subepithelial connective tissue grafts in the treatment of gingival recessions, *Journal of Periodontology*, 72(11): 1470–1476.

[30] Goaslind G, Roberston P, Mahan C et al. (1977). Thickness of facial gingiva, *Journal of Periodontology*, 48(12): 768–771.

[31] Mörmann W., Schaer F., Firestone A. R. (1981). The relationship between success of free gingival grafts and transplant thickness revascularization and shrinkage a one-year clinical study. *Journal of Periodontology*, 52(2): 74-80.

[32] Silverstein L. H., Kurtzman D., Garnick J. J., Trager P. S., Waters P. K. (1994). Connective tissue grafting for improved implant esthetics: clinical technique. *Implant Dentistry,* 3(4): 231-234.

[33] Moghaddas H., Ghasemi N. (1999). Comparison of the palatal connective tissue graft as a membrane with and without hydroxyapatite in the treatment of infrabony defects. *Shahid Beheshti Dental Journal,* 17: 60-68.

[34] Mitrano T. I., Grob M. S., Carrión F., et al. (2010) Culture and characterization of mesenchymal stem cells from human gingival tissue. *Journal of Periodontology,* 81(6): 917-925.

[35] Esfahanian V., Golestaneh H., Moghaddas O., Ghafari M. R. Efficacy of connective tissue with and without periosteum in regeneration of intrabony defects. *Journal of Dental Research Dental Clinics Dental Prospects,* 8(4): 189-196.

[36] Newman Michael G., Takei Henry H. and Carranza Fermin A. *Carranza's clinical periodontology.* Philadelphia: W. B. Saunders Co, 2007.

[37] Staffileno H., Levy S., Gargiulo A. (1966). Histologic study of cellular mobilization and repair following a periosteal retention operation via split thickness mucogingival flap surger. *Journal of Periodontology*, 37(2): 117-131.

[38] Gargiulo A. W., Arrocha R. (1967). Histo-clinical evaluation of free gingival grafts. *Periodontics,* 5(6): 285-291.

[39] Janson W. A., Ruben M. P., Kraamer G. M., et al. (1969). Development of the blood supply to split-thickness free gingival autografts. *Journal of Periodontology*, 40(12): 707.

[40] Caffesse R. G., Carraro J. J., Carranza F. A. (1972). Injertos givgivales libres en perros: estudio clinico e histologico [Free givgival grafts in dogs: clinical and histological study]. *Revista de la Asoiacion Odontologica Argentina* 60: 465.

[41] Oliver R. C., Löe H., Karring T. (1968). Microscopic evaluation of the healing and revascularization of free gingival grafts. *Journal of Periodontology*, 3(2): 84-95.

[42] Gordon H. P., Sullivan H. C., Atkins J. H. (1968). Free autogenous gingival grafts. Part II. Supplemental findings: histology of the graft site. *Periodontics,* 6(3): 130-133.

[43] Petrungaro P. (2001) Using platelet rich plasma to accelerate soft tissue maturation in esthetic periodontal surgery. *Compendium of Continuing Education in Dentistry,* 22(9): 729-736.

[44] Langer L., Langer B. Mucogingival Surgery: Esthetic Treatment of Gingival Recession. Clinical Application. In (Wilson TG, Kornman KS, Newman MG, eds. *Advances in Periodontics.* Hanover Park, IL: Quintessence, 1992), 248-260.

In: Connective Tissue
Editor: Jim M. Pearson

ISBN: 978-1-53617-875-3
© 2020 Nova Science Publishers, Inc.

Chapter 3

SUBEPITHELIAL CONNECTIVE TISSUE GRAFTS (SCTGS) IN PERIODONTOLOGY

Aysan Lektemur Alpan[1,*] *and Nebi Cansin Karakan*[2]
[1]Periodontology, Pamukkale University, Denizli, Turkey
[2]Periodontology, Afyonkarahisar Health Sciences University, Afyonkarahisar, Turkey

ABSTRACT

Periodontal plastic surgery applications have increased in modern dentistry as the importance of patients to their appearance. For this purpose, many techniques and flap designs have been used to treat gingival recession, but subepithelial connective tissue graft (SCTG) seems to be the gold standard procedure. SCTGs can be harvested from several areas in the mouth such as maxillary tuberosity and palate with different approaches which can affect graft quality and postoperative complications. In this section, rationale of SCTG, harvesting techniques, clinical success and possible postoperative complications will be discussed in the light of literature.

---

* Corresponding Author's E-mail: ysnlpn@gmail.com.

Keywords: autogenous grafts, autografts, dental implants, gingival recession, periodontal, plastic surgery, soft tissue grafting, subepithelial connective tissue

INTRODUCTION

For various reasons, patients may present loss of gingival tissue, which can negatively affect esthetics and function. In recent years, clinicians and researchers have shown increasing interest in mucogingival surgery to reconstruct the soft tissue around the teeth and implants. The term 'Periodontal Plastic Surgery', was suggested by Miller in 1993 [1], and accepted in modern periodontology to define 'surgical procedures performed to prevent or correct anatomic, developmental, traumatic or disease-induced defects of the gingiva, alveolar mucosa or bone' [2]. The main indications for root coverage procedures are aesthetic requests, treatment of tooth sensitivity and increased keratinized tissue to reduce the risk of defect progression [3]. The clinical objective of the root coverage procedure is coverage of root completely; this means a location of the gingival margin to cemento-enamel junction (CEJ) that no longer has a probing depth and without inflammation [3].

Autologous subgingival connective tissue graft (SCTG) is an essential therapeutic tool for functional and aesthetic mucogingival periodontal surgery and implantology. SCTG usage was first described by Edel in 1974 [4], since then it has continued to develop in terms of technical indications, usage indications and harvesting methods. Root coverage [5], increasing the height and thickness of keratinized mucosa [6], papilla reconstruction [7], peri-implant soft tissue augmentation [8] and alveolar ridge preservation [9] are the main usage areas of SCTG in periodontology. Although SCTG is often harvested from palate, maxillary tuberosity and vestıbular gingiva of existing teeth can be used as donor site [10]. The graft can be obtained in various harvesting techniques. Donor site localization can affect the shape, volume and thickness of graft thus graft reshaping must be necessary to adapt it into recipient site [10]. In this chapter, the procedures for harvesting of SCTG's, their use, possible complications and clinical success of SCTG were evaluated.

HISTOLOGIC CONTENT OF SCTG

The main components of the subepithelial connective tissue are collagen fibers (approximately 60% by volume), fibroblasts (5%), matrix, nerves and vessels (approximately 35%). The connective tissue in the gingiva is known as *lamina propria* and reveals a structure that has two layers: 1) *papillary layer* subjacent to the epithelium and includes papillary projections between the epithelium rete pegs. 2) *Reticular layer* is located above the periosteum of the alveolar bone. Connective tissue consists of cellular and extracellular components which are composed of ground substance and fibers. The ground substance fills the space between cells and fibers. It is amorphous and contains high rate of water. It includes proteoglycans, mainly hyaluronic acid and chondroitin sulfate, and glycoproteins, mainly fibronectin. Connective tissue fibers are collagen, reticular and elastic. Fibroblast is the main cellular element in the connective tissue and fibroblasts play a key role in the development, maintenance and repair of the connective tissue [11].

CLINICAL USAGE OF SCTG IN PERIODONTOLOGY

Periodontal plastic procedures involve a range of surgical techniques aimed at achieving improvements in what is called nowadays the pink esthetic. In addition to achieving satisfactory results, these procedures attempt to obtain some balance between function and aesthetics. Furthermore, the need for performing aesthetics became more and more important as implant rehabilitation became widespread [12]. The aim of plastic periodontal procedures is to prevent and correct anatomical, developmental, traumatic or plaque-induced defects of the gingiva as well as alveolar mucosa or bone [13].

Different techniques either with a SCTG or other graft substitutes have been used for treating gingival recessions, such as the coronally advanced flap (CAF), laterally positional flap, semilunar flap, tunnel technique or the VISTA technique [3, 14, 15]. It was suggested that a minimum of 2 mm keratinized tissue (KT) is needed to prevent recession if plaque control is suboptimal [16].

Among this techniques SCTG has been proposed as a means of increasing the amount of root coverage obtained by a CAF (Figure 1). Case reports of this combination have been published in natural teeth, non-carious cervical lesion teeth and implants [17-19]. SCTG has been suggested to act as a biological filler that improves flap-root adaptation and stability during early wound repair [20]. As a result, the gingival phenotype becomes thicker and has a higher chance of gaining full root coverage [21] (Figures 2, 3). The results of the meta-analyzes revealed that the use of SCTG provided a statistically significant reduction in gingival recession (GR) and gain in KT, especially when compared to guided tissue regeneration (GTR) procedures [22, 23]. Additionally, in a systematic review SCTG was emphasized as the 'gold standard' procedure in the treatment of recession-type defects [24]. According to results of a systematic review that included fifteen randomized control studies, CAF+SCTG could maintain long-term stability and result in better long-term efficacy of root coverage than CAF alone [25].

Extensive evidence reports positive outcomes of SCTG following the root coverage procedures in the treatment of single gingival recessions, whilst studies are currently available reporting the outcomes for the treatment of multiple gingival recessions. A systematic review included 4 articles [26] evaluated the results collected with different root-coverage procedures in the treatment of multiple recession type defects. According to their results all periodontal plastic surgery procedures (i.e., CAF alone or in combination with SCTG) provided benefits in recession depth, clinical attachment level and width of KT. In a 5 years of follow-up trial compared the clinical outcomes of CAF alone with those of CAF+SCTG in the treatment of multiple gingival recessions. No statistically significant difference between CAF+SCTG and CAF alone was reported in terms of recession reduction and complete root coverage in 6 months but in 5 years slight coronal shift of the gingival margin named 'creeping attachment' occurred in the CAF+SCTG group while slight apical reposition of the margins in CAF group [27]. A randomized controlled trial performed in multiple gingival recessions, compared short-term (6 months and 1 year) and long-term (5 years) clinical and esthetic outcomes of the CAF that of CAF+SCTG. According the study results CAF+SCTG was linked with an increased chance of obtaining complete root coverage at 5 years [28].

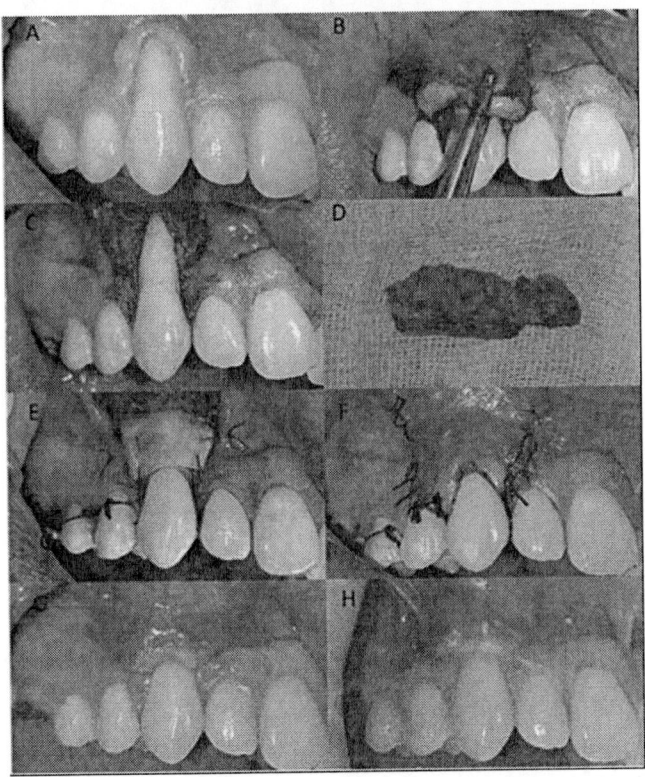

Figure 1. Coronally advanced flap combined with SCTG in the treatment of Miller Class II gingival recession. A- Right canine tooth with GR; B-Flap prepared and released; C-Root planning was performed; D-Harvested SCTG; E-SCTG placed on root surface; F-Flap was placed coronally; G, H- Postoperative view.

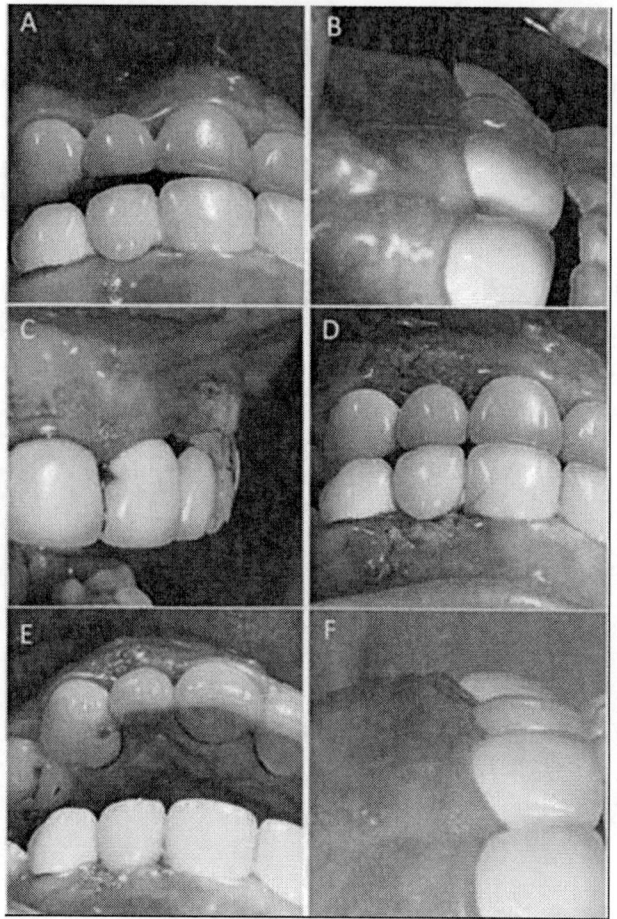

Figure 2. Soft tissue contour augmentation. A, B-Right lateral tooth area with bone and soft tissue deficiency; C, D- Pedicle connective tissue was used to provide soft tissue contour; E, F- Postoperative view.

Surgical treatment of multiple Class III-V recession defects is seemed to be more complicated comparing Class I-II Miller recessions, because of the loss of papilla and interdental bone which must be provide recipient bed and blood supply for the graft. Mercado et al. [29] investigated the effect of SCTG with or without enamel matrix derivative (EMD) application in a long term clinical trial. They founded EMD+SCTG more effective than only SCTG in terms of gaining KT, closing GR even reducing the pain at donor site ($p < 0.01$).

Subepithelial Connective Tissue Grafts (SCTGs) in Periodontology 119

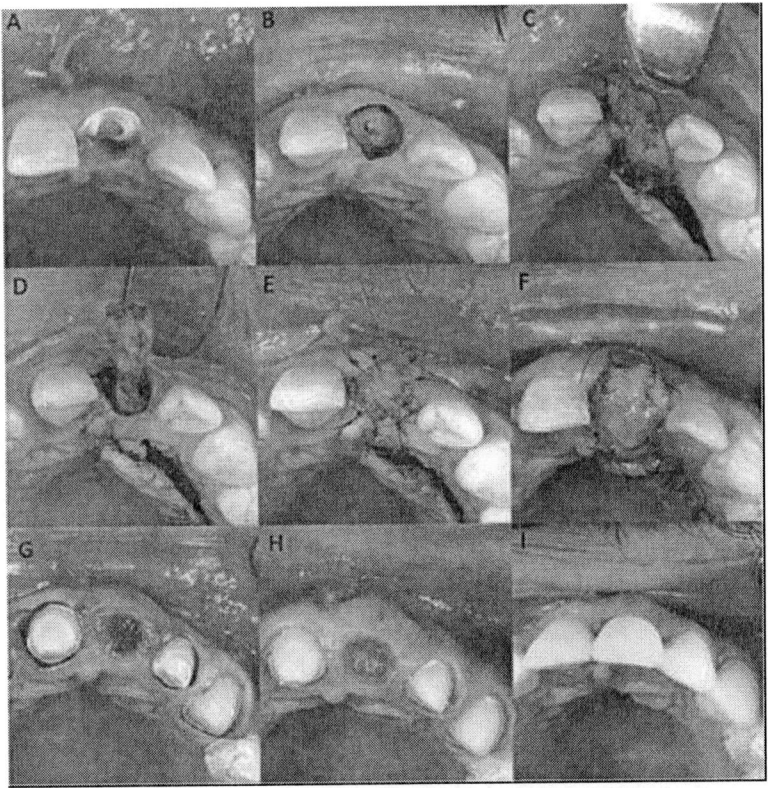

Figure 3. Socket preservation with SCTG A, B- Preoperative view; C, D- Pedicle SCTG was obtained; E, F- SCTG was placed; G, H- Healing pattern; I- Final prosthesis and gained tissue volume.

The tunnel procedure for obtaining root coverage was introduced in 1994 and termed the supraperiosteal envelope technique [30, 31]. With this procedure, the interdental papilla remains intact and SCTG which does not need to be completely covered placed in this tunnel. Not covering the graft completely creates an advantage to gain additional KT, but as a disadvantage exposed tissue might not be an exact color match. The technique is minimally invasive and reduces postoperative discomfort at the recipient site (Figures 4, 5). Recently, the tunnel technique was modified named modified tunnel technique to include coronal positioning of the marginal tissue for covering all SCTG [32]. In a RCT, the efficacy of a modified tunnel+ SCTG technique in the treatment of multiple Class

III gingival recessions. According to their data modified tunnel/SCTG technique is predictable for the treatment of multiple class III recession-type defects [33]. Root coverage rate of this technique varies between 84% and 96% [30, 34-36].

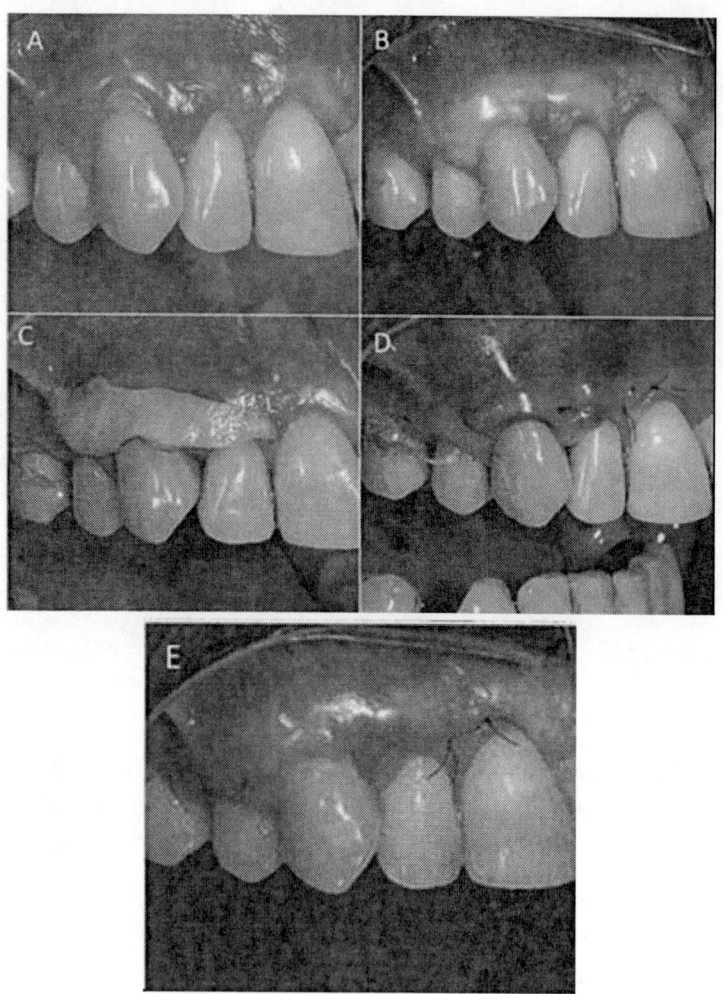

Figure 4. Images using SCTG in tunnel technique. A-Miller Class I gingival recession in right lower incisor tooth; B- postoperative 1-month view of operated area; C- Measuring SCTG according to recession site; D- Placing SCTG into tunnel and suturing the area; E- Postoperative 10 days.

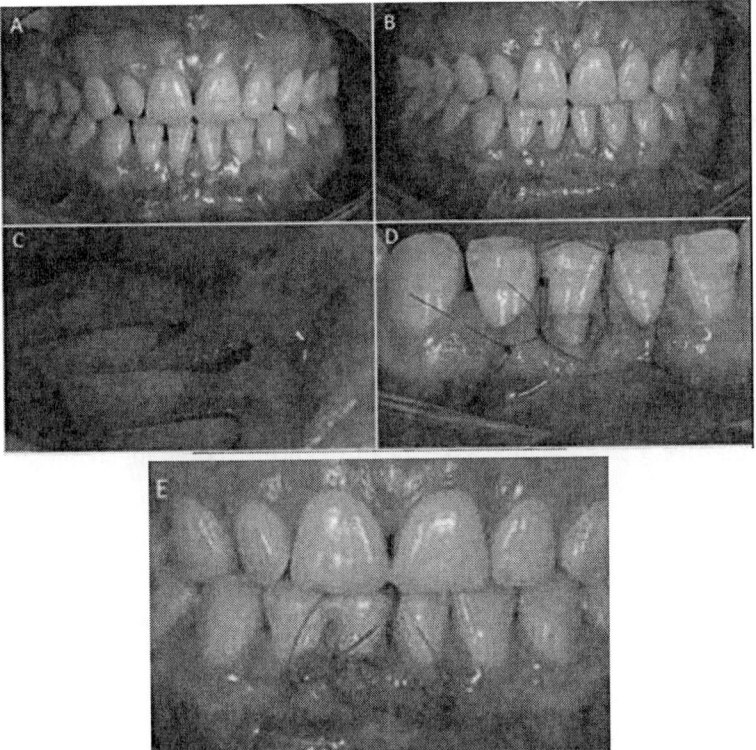

Figure 5. Images using SCTG in tunnel techique. A-Miller Class I gingival recession in right lower incisor tooth, B- postoperative 1 month view of operated area, C- Creating a tunnel in relevant area, D- Placing SCTG in tunnel and suturing the area, E- Healing in 10 days.

Clinicians may think about the use of autogenous soft tissue grafts to improve peri-implant soft tissue health or prevent marginal bone levels in implant sites in the presence of insufficient soft tissue. When it is desired to increase soft tissue thickness at implant sites, clinicians should consider SCTG procedures to provide greater stability at interproximal marginal bone levels [37]. Two different methods can be applied to strengthen the peri-implant soft tissue [38]:

1. KT width enlargement using an apically positioned flap/vestibuloplasty (in combination with a free gingival graft (FGG) or an allogeneic or xenogenic graft material).

2. Soft tissue volume gain with the help of a SCTG or soft tissue replacement grafts.

Recent systematic reviews concluded that an inadequate peri-implant KT was associated with greater plaque deposition, inflammation symptoms, recession of soft tissue, and loss of attachment [39-41].

In a consensus statement; it was suggested that to increase mucosal thickness at implant site using immediate or delayed placement of SCTG in terms of clinical indications included a prevention of mucosal recessions/compensation of volume deficiencies and facilitation of tissue adaptation at implant placement for functional and/or aesthetic purposes can improve peri-implant tissue health. Furthermore, thickening of the mucosa with the help of SCTG did not changed in plaque index, bleeding on probing or probing depth as compared to control. Significantly higher interproximal marginal bone levels were obtained after the application of SCTG when compared to controls [42]. Treating peri-implant soft tissue defects with SCTG is highly recommended, regardless of KT width or thickness. Autogenous graft substitutes are often used for increasing tissue thickness and minimizing the post-operative mucosal recession during immediate implant placement or at the time of implant uncovering [43].

Table 1. SCTG indications

Intension healing (primary or secondary)	Indication
Primary	Root coverage [44, 45]
	Peri-implant soft tissue thickness Augmentation [46, 47]
	Immediate implant placement [48, 49]
	Peri-implant soft tissue dehiscence [50, 51]
Secondary	Ridge augmentation [9]

SCTG HARVESTING TECHNIQUES

Techniques can be identified in five main titles.

Single Incision Technique

In this technique a single incision is made approximately 2mm below the teeth at the palatal region. The incision length is depending on the amount of gingival recession and the extent of SCTG which we would like to harvest. This technique is least painful and traumatic harvesting method. The first incision is made at 90 degrees to the long axis of the teeth until the bone contact is ensured thereafter the second incision is made beneath the epithelial layer to separate the epithelium from the connective tissue. Afterwards third incision is performed to separate the connective tissue from the periosteal layer [52-54] (Figure 6).

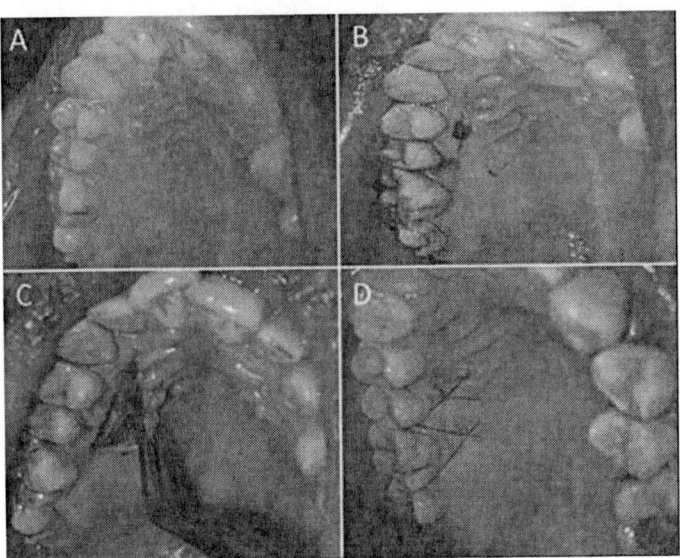

Figure 6. SCTG harvesting using single insicion technique. A- Palate, B- A single insicion extending canine to molar, C- Separating SCTG from periost, D- Suturing the area using mattress sutures.

Modified Single Incision Technique

This technique differs from the single incision technique at the point that we focus on to raise a partial thickness flap when making the first incision. This first incision is performed far apically as required. The thickness of the flap should be sufficient to prevent or reduce the tearing and sloughing risk. Following this the second incision is made at 90 degrees to the long axis of the teeth until the bone contact is ensured. At this point we can specify that the incision order is reversed when compared to the single incision technique. Afterwards the connective tissue layer is raised from bone via periosteal elevator. Two vertical and one horizontal incisions is performed beneath the flap ensuring bone contact to separate it from the underlying bone. Vertical incisions are positioned at the mesial and distal edge of the flap and horizontal incision is beneath the first incision line at the apical edge of the connective tissue. Special blades called the 'Barraquer cataract knives' and 'AVS blade' can be used to make vertical and horizontal incisions. The 'Barraquer cataract knives' are used in opthalmic operations. These blades are sharp, thin and long enough to make incisions and release the graft from bone at the mesial and distal edges. The space beneath the partial thickness flap is limited, therefore maneuvering of the normal Bard-Parker blade No. 11 or 15 becomes difficult and can lead to tearing of the overlying partial thickness flap. For this reason, 'barraquer knives' can be used in SCTG operations. In the medial incisions 'AVS blade' can also be used depending on the difficulties of the surgery region [55].

Trap Door Technique

Trap door technique includes two vertical incisions and one horizontal incision. Horizontal incision is made 2 mm under the teeth similar to single incision and modified single incision. Parallel vertical incisions are performed at the mesial and distal edge of the operation region. The length of these two incisions depends on the amount of SCTG which we would like to harvest. Also the space between these two parallel vertical incisions depends on the same subject. After making incisions a partial thickness flap is raised via Bard-Parker blade no. 15 and afterwards a supraperiosteal incision is made to release the connective tissue graft. Finally a medial incision is made to separate the graft from palatal gingiva [4, 56].

SCTG Harvesting with Free Gingival Graft

Zucchelli and coworkers introduced the de-epithelialized gingival graft [44]. In this technique the graft is derived as free gingival graft from palatal gingiva which is de-epithelialized extraorally by surgical blades. Two vertical and two horizontal incisions are performed with approximately 1.5-2 mm deep. The length of the incisions and size of the graft depends on the recipient area. When the free gingival graft is harvested, then de-epithelialized extraorally by surgical blades carefully. It should be ensured that there is no residual epithelial layer over the graft. The donor site is left for healing by second intention. This is an important disadvantage of this technique [57, 58].

SCTG from Maxillary Tuberosity

In this technique distal wedge procedure can be performed [59] or gingival cuff can be harvested and extraoral de-epithelialization is performed. Distal wedge operation allows primary closure. Nevertheless performing gingivectomy and extraoral de-epithelialization technique can be easier [60]. Recently a punch (Nizam punch) which composed of two sharp punches and a shank was fabricated to obtain SCTG from maxillary tuberosity. This punch was designed especially in using peri-implant KT augmentation. Minimal tissue loss in the donor site and easy use are advantages of this technique, but the need to have a thick gum in the tuberosity region is a disadvantage of this technique [10].

ADVANTAGES AND DISADVANTAGES OF SCTG HARVESTING TECHNIQUES

The single incision or modified single incision technique seems to be the best method according to the primary closure of the donor site among the palatal region harvesting techniques. Adequate blood supply depending on avoiding vertical incisions and easy suturing are advantages of the single incision techniques. However performing this surgical method is more difficult than the others and reduced visibility is a disadvantage [55, 57]. When we compare the single incision and modified single incision techniques, in modified single incision technique first incision is focused on raising partial thickness flap, thus we can preserve soft tissue integrity at first and more visible operation site due to less bleeding may be seen as an advantage [57].

Trap door technique provides better sight of the donor site but afterwards suturing and primary closuring the donor site is more difficult than the single incision techniques. Blood supply may be jeopardized by vertical incisions and risk of sloughing is critical [4].

In harvesting SCTG with free gingival graft we need an extraoral second step of surgery that is used to separate the epithelium layer from the connective tissue. In addition to this magnification is very important to perform extraoral de-epithelialization of the graft in the above mentioned second step of surgery in the SCTG harvesting with free gingival graft technique. Also the secondary healing of the donor site is a disadvantage of this method [44, 61]. In SCTG harvesting with free gingival graft technique it has been suggested that optimum de-epithelialization of the free gingival graft is important. Harvested SCTG should include mainly *lamina propria* but not the glandular tissue [44]. In a recent systematic review and meta-analysis, coronally advanced flap with conventional SCTG or SCTG with de-epithelialized gingival graft harvesting techniques have been compared and de-epithelialized gingival graft revealed slightly meaner root coverage than SCTG at 1-year follow-up. Mean root coverage is 89.3% in the SCTG studies is and 94% in the de-epithelialized gingival graft studies [58].

Table 2. SCTG harvesting techniques

Author	Technique
Edel (1974)	Trap Door Technique: As described above a primary incision is made parallel to the long axis of the teeth. Thereafter two parallel vertical incisions are performed. Then flap is raised and the SCTG is harvested.
Raetzke (1985)	Two converging crescent shaped horizontal incisions are made. Afterwards flap is raised and SCTG is harvested. SCTG includes epithelial collar.
Harris (1992)	Graft knife technique/Harris double-blade technique: This method is a modification of Trap Door Technique. The difference is split thickness flap is raised and the SCTG is harvested via a special graft blade.
Bruno (1994)	Double incision technique: Two parallel and horizontal incisions are made contacting bone. Then a full thickness flap is raised to harvest the flap.
Hürzeler and Weng (1999)	Single incision technique: A single horizontal incision is made contacting the underlying bone. Afterwards a split thickness flap is raised. Vertical incisions and releasing medial incision are performed beneath the flap and SCTG is harvested.
Lorenzana and Allen (2000)	Similar to Hürzeler and Weng's single incision technique. Instead of the vertical and medial releasing incisions manipulation of the SCTG with Corn suture pilers or other delicate tissue forceps are necessary to harvest the graft.
Del Pizzo et al. (2002)	An extended horizontal single incision is performed until contacting the bone. Split thickness flap is raised. When harvesting the graft, periosteum should be leaven on the bone to accelerate the wound healing in the donor region.
Ribeiro et al. (2008)	Split SCTG technique: A single incision technique is performed to harvest the graft from palatal region. SCTG should be in maximum thickness to split it cross-sectional way. The SCTG is not divided into two parts, but the length of the SCTG is approximately two fold longer than the primarily harvested graft.
McLeod et al. (2009)	A back action periodontal surgical chisel is used to de-epithelialize the palatal donor region. Afterwards similar to harvest free gingival graft, SCTG is harvested keeping the periosteum and a little amount of connective tissue

Table 2. (Continued)

Author	Technique
Zuchelli et al. (2010)	Two horizontal (the coronal incision was performed 1–1.5 mm apical to the soft tissue margin of the adjacent teeth) and two vertical incisions were performed to obtain a free gingival graft. The fatty tissue (yellow in color) was eliminated. The graft was de-epithelialized with a 15c blade.
Bosco and Bosco (2017)	A split thickness flap is raised while keeping periosteum on the bone. The graft is harvested consisting of epithelium. Then extraoral bisection is made. One graft includes only the connective tissue while the other one consists of the epithelial layer in addition to the connective tissue. The epithelial graft is repositioned at the donor site similar to a free gingival graft.

We can either receive SCTG from anterior palatal region or posterior lateral palatal region. It depends on the thickness of the soft tissue and anatomic factors. Rarely if the dentition ends with first molar teeth in the upper jaw, we can also harvest the SCTG from maxillary tuberosity. In the presence of second and third molars this method can be difficult to perform. We can receive the graft but less extensive SCTG can be harvested [60, 62]. Maxillary tuberosity SCTG tissue has high amount of *lamina propria*, consequently connective tissue fibers and low amount of adipose tissue and submucosa [59]. Higher amounts of submucosa tissue in the graft may cause graft shrinkage, less soft tissue volume gain and minimal or no effect on epithelium keratinization [59, 63]. It has been reported that *lamina propria* includes adequate amount of cells, vessels and fibers to provide sufficient tissue thickness to cover the gingival recessions with fine aesthetic outcomes [64]. Therefore SCTG from maxillary tuberosity can be a fine option when comparing to SCTG which is harvested from palatal region [65]. In a randomized controlled clinical study, around single tooth implants there has been no significant difference between maxillary tuberosity SCTG and SCTG harvested from lateral palate in volume gain, however significantly higher keratinized tissue width has been observed in maxillary tuberosity SCTG group [63]. It has been reported that SCTG from maxillary tuberosity with ring technique via punch can be an alternative method to increase soft tissue volume around the dental implants. In this method ring shaped SCTG is harvested via punch from donor area [10].

SCTG LIMITATIONS

Patient morbidity has been reported as one of the most important deficiencies of the autologous soft tissue graft procedure [66]. Although necrosis of graft and palatal site, pain and excessive hemorrhage, protracted discomfort, increased chances of infection, also sometimes loss of sensation may occur as complications of SCTG in donor site [67]. Postsurgical swelling and ecchymosis, external root resorption, gingival cysts, gingival abscess, exostosis, loss of graft, epithelial cell discharge, tunnel like defects in gingiva may be observed as recipient site complications [67]. In some reasons SCTG operations may not produce the desired result. Insufficient height of interdental bone, reflection of all interdental papilla, horizontal incision placed apical to CEJ, flap penetration, graft that is too thick or too thin, tension in graft, ineffective postsurgical biofilm control during healing, inadequate height and thickness of keratinized tissue some of the reasons for failure of operation [43, 67]. Some techniques have been tried for reducing postoperative complications in donor site. In a study authors placed platelet rich fibrin (PRF) in SCTG donor site and according to their results, PRF reduced postoperative complications, pain measured using visual analogue scale and analgesic intake also provided better color match and healing measured by early healing index (EHI) [68]. Stavropoulou et al. [69] compared cyanoacrylates tissue adhesive and polytetrafluoroethylene (PTFE) suture efficacy in the SCTG donor site. At the end of the study they did not found a statistical significance in terms of EHI, postoperative pain and analgesic intake. Additive EMD in donor site in palate reduced postoperative pain at 2nd, 7th and 14th days postoperatively comparing the control group which had no additional implementation [29]. Relevant studies are ongoing, but no gold standard has yet been established to prevent postoperative complications.

Prolonged intraoperative and postoperative bleeding caused by the palatal vessels' injury is also one of the complications of soft tissue harvesting [70]. In order to reduce this complication, palatine area anatomy should be known. The anatomy of the palatal vault affects the risk of damaging the greater palatine artery (GPA). In one study, the distance of the artery was found to be 7 mm in the shallow palate, 12 mm in the average palate and 17 mm in high palate from CEJ [71]. Monnet-Corti et al. found that the average distance from the GPA to the canines and second molars was 12.07 ± 2.9 mm and 14.7 ± 2.9 mm, respectively [72]. A recent systematic review focused on this, according to their results the location of the greater palatine foremen (GPF) located 0.84% between first and second molar; 6.21% midpalatal aspect of second molar; 21.25% between second and third molar; 57.08% midpalatal aspect of third molar and 13.54% distal to third molar. The distance from the GPA to the CEJ was found as follows: 13.9 ± 1 mm to the second molar, 13.0 ± 2.4 mm to the first molar, 13.8 ± 2.1 mm to the second premolar, 11.8 ± 2.2 mm to the first premolar, and 9.9 ± 2.9 mm to the canine [73]. Safety zone is presented in Figure 7.

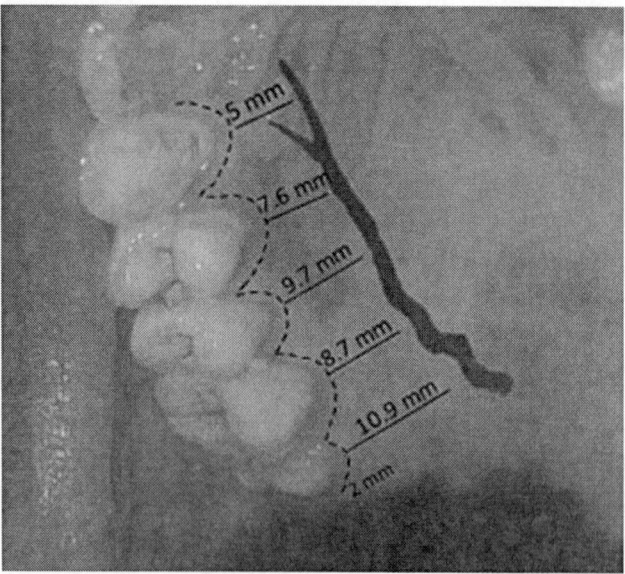

Figure 7. Safety distance to harvest SCTG from palate without harming GPA.

Conclusion

The distinctive nature of connective tissue is still the most reliable and gold standard technique for the treatment of various soft tissue augmentation surgeries, especially single gingival recessions. The use of SCTG in the treatment of gingival recessions has increased significantly in periodontal plastic surgery with high success rates. With the increase in use, many techniques have been proposed and used to make the SCTG harvesting procedure easier, less traumatic and more predictable.

Acknowledgments

We would like to thank Dr. Olcay BAKAR for sharing his cases with us.

References

[1] Miller, P. D., Jr. (1993). "Root coverage grafting for regeneration and aesthetics" *Periodontol 2000* 1 (1). 118-27.

[2] Wennstrom, J. L. (1996). "Mucogingival therapy" *Ann Periodontol* 1 (1). 671-701.

[3] Cairo, F. (2017). "Periodontal plastic surgery of gingival recessions at single and multiple teeth" *Periodontol 2000* 75 (1). 296-316.

[4] Edel, A. (1974). "Clinical evaluation of free connective tissue grafts used to increase the width of keratinised gingiva" *J Clin Periodontol* 1 (4). 185-96.

[5] Nizam, N., Bengisu, O., Sonmez, S. (2015). "Micro- and macrosurgical techniques in the coverage of gingival recession using connective tissue graft: 2 years follow-up" *J Esthet Restor Dent* 27 (2). 71-83.

[6] Wessel, J. R., Tatakis, D. N. (2008). "Patient outcomes following subepithelial connective tissue graft and free gingival graft procedures" *J Periodontol* 79 (3). 425-30.

[7] Nemcovsky, C. E. (2001). "Interproximal papilla augmentation procedure: a novel surgical approach and clinical evaluation of 10 consecutive procedures" *Int J Periodontics Restorative Dent* 21 (6). 553-9.

[8] Santagata, M., Tartaro, G., D'Amato, S. (2015). "Clinical and histologic comparative study of subepithelial connective tissue graft and extracellular matrix membrane. A preliminary split-mouth study in humans" *Int J Periodontics Restorative Dent* 35 (1). 85-91.

[9] Akcali, A., Schneider, D., Unlu, F., Bicakci, N., Kose, T., Hammerle, C. H. (2015). "Soft tissue augmentation of ridge defects in the maxillary anterior area using two different methods: a randomized controlled clinical trial" *Clin Oral Implants Res* 26 (6). 688-95.

[10] Nizam, N., Akcali, A. (2019). "A Novel Connective Tissue Graft Harvesting Technique: The Ring Method" *Int J Periodontics Restorative Dent* 39 (3). 422-429.

[11] Embery, G., Waddington, R. J., Hall, R. C., Last, K. S. (2000). "Connective tissue elements as diagnostic aids in periodontology" *Periodontol 2000* 24 193-214.

[12] Novaes, A. B., Jr., Palioto, D. B. (2019). "Experimental and clinical studies on plastic periodontal procedures" *Periodontol 2000* 79 (1). 56-80.

[13] Miller, P. D., Jr. (1988). "Regenerative and reconstructive periodontal plastic surgery. Mucogingival surgery" *Dent Clin North Am* 32 (2). 287-306.

[14] Stefanini, M., Marzadori, M., Aroca, S., Felice, P., Sangiorgi, M., Zucchelli, G. (2018). "Decision making in root-coverage procedures for the esthetic outcome" *Periodontol 2000* 77 (1). 54-64.

[15] Zadeh, H. H. (2011). "Minimally invasive treatment of maxillary anterior gingival recession defects by vestibular incision subperiosteal tunnel access and platelet-derived growth factor BB" *Int J Periodontics Restorative Dent* 31 (6). 653-60.

[16] Scheyer, E. T., Sanz, M., Dibart, S., Greenwell, H., John, V., Kim, D. M., Langer, L., Neiva, R., Rasperini, G. (2015). "Periodontal soft tissue non-root coverage procedures: a consensus report from the AAP Regeneration Workshop" *J Periodontol* 86 (2 Suppl). S73-6.

[17] Martorelli de Lima, A. F., da Silva, R. C., Joly, J. C., Tatakis, D. N. (2006). "Coronally positioned flap with subepithelial connective tissue graft for root coverage: various indications and flap designs" *J Int Acad Periodontol* 8 (2). 53-60.

[18] Deliberador, T. M., Bosco, A. F., Martins, T. M., Nagata, M. J. (2009). "Treatment of gingival recessions associated to cervical abrasion lesions with subepithelial connective tissue graft: a case report" *Eur J Dent* 3 (4). 318-23.

[19] Shibli, J. A., d'avila, S., Marcantonio, E., Jr. (2004). "Connective tissue graft to correct peri-implant soft tissue margin: A clinical report" *J Prosthet Dent* 91 (2). 119-22.

[20] Cairo, F., Cortellini, P., Pilloni, A., Nieri, M., Cincinelli, S., Amunni, F., Pagavino, G., Tonetti, M. S. (2016). "Clinical efficacy of coronally advanced flap with or without connective tissue graft for the treatment of multiple adjacent gingival recessions in the aesthetic area: a randomized controlled clinical trial" *J Clin Periodontol* 43 (10). 849-56.

[21] Rebele, S. F., Zuhr, O., Schneider, D., Jung, R. E., Hurzeler, M. B. (2014). "Tunnel technique with connective tissue graft versus coronally advanced flap with enamel matrix derivative for root coverage: a RCT using 3D digital measuring methods. Part II. Volumetric studies on healing dynamics and gingival dimensions" *J Clin Periodontol* 41 (6). 593-603.

[22] Zucchelli, G., Clauser, C., De Sanctis, M., Calandriello, M. (1998). "Mucogingival versus guided tissue regeneration procedures in the treatment of deep recession type defects" *J Periodontol* 69 (2). 138-45.

[23] Tatakis, D. N., Trombelli, L. (2000). "Gingival recession treatment: guided tissue regeneration with bioabsorbable membrane versus connective tissue graft" *J Periodontol* 71 (2). 299-307.

[24] Chambrone, L., Chambrone, D., Pustiglioni, F. E., Chambrone, L. A., Lima, L. A. (2008). "Can subepithelial connective tissue grafts be considered the gold standard procedure in the treatment of Miller Class I and II recession-type defects?" *J Dent* 36 (9). 659-71.

[25] Dai, A., Huang, J. P., Ding, P. H., Chen, L. L. (2019). "Long-term stability of root coverage procedures for single gingival recessions: A systematic review and meta-analysis" *J Clin Periodontol* 46 (5). 572-585.

[26] Chambrone, L., Lima, L. A., Pustiglioni, F. E., Chambrone, L. A. (2009). "Systematic review of periodontal plastic surgery in the treatment of multiple recession-type defects" *J Can Dent Assoc* 75 (3). 203a-203f.

[27] Pini-Prato, G. P., Cairo, F., Nieri, M., Franceschi, D., Rotundo, R., Cortellini, P. (2010). "Coronally advanced flap versus connective tissue graft in the treatment of multiple gingival recessions: a split-mouth study with a 5-year follow-up" *J Clin Periodontol* 37 (7). 644-50.

[28] Zucchelli, G., Mounssif, I., Mazzotti, C., Stefanini, M., Marzadori, M., Petracci, E., Montebugnoli, L. (2014). "Coronally advanced flap with and without connective tissue graft for the treatment of multiple gingival recessions: a comparative short- and long-term controlled randomized clinical trial" *J Clin Periodontol* 41 (4). 396-403.

[29] Mercado, F., Hamlet, S., Ivanovski, S. (2019). "Sub-epithelial connective tissue graft with or without enamel matrix derivative for the treatment of multiple Class III-IV recessions in lower anterior teeth: a 3-year randomized clinical trial" *J Periodontol.*

[30] Allen, A. L. (1994). "Use of the supraperiosteal envelope in soft tissue grafting for root coverage. II. Clinical results" *Int J Periodontics Restorative Dent* 14 (4). 302-15.

[31] Allen, A. L. (1994). "Use of the supraperiosteal envelope in soft tissue grafting for root coverage. I. Rationale and technique" *Int J Periodontics Restorative Dent* 14 (3). 216-27.

[32] Zucchelli, G., Mounssif, I. (2015). "Periodontal plastic surgery" *Periodontol 2000* 68 (1). 333-68.

[33] Aroca, S., Keglevich, T., Nikolidakis, D., Gera, I., Nagy, K., Azzi, R., Etienne, D. (2010). "Treatment of class III multiple gingival recessions: a randomized-clinical trial" *J Clin Periodontol* 37 (1). 88-97.

[34] Zabalegui, I., Sicilia, A., Cambra, J., Gil, J., Sanz, M. (1999). "Treatment of multiple adjacent gingival recessions with the tunnel subepithelial connective tissue graft: a clinical report" *Int J Periodontics Restorative Dent* 19 (2). 199-206.

[35] Tozum, T. F., Dini, F. M. (2003). "Treatment of adjacent gingival recessions with subepithelial connective tissue grafts and the modified tunnel technique" *Quintessence Int* 34 (1). 7-13.

[36] Tozum, T. F., Keceli, H. G., Guncu, G. N., Hatipoglu, H., Sengun, D. (2005). "Treatment of gingival recession: comparison of two techniques of subepithelial connective tissue graft" *J Periodontol* 76 (11). 1842-8.

[37] Thoma, D. S., Naenni, N., Figuero, E., Hammerle, C. H. F., Schwarz, F., Jung, R. E., Sanz-Sanchez, I. (2018). "Effects of soft tissue augmentation procedures on peri-implant health or disease: A systematic review and meta-analysis" *Clin Oral Implants Res* 29 Suppl 15 32-49.

[38] Bassetti, R. G., Stahli, A., Bassetti, M. A., Sculean, A. (2017). "Soft tissue augmentation around osseointegrated and uncovered dental implants: a systematic review" *Clin Oral Investig* 21 (1). 53-70.

[39] Wennstrom, J. L., Derks, J. (2012). "Is there a need for keratinized mucosa around implants to maintain health and tissue stability?" *Clin Oral Implants Res* 23 Suppl 6 136-46.

[40] Brito, C., Tenenbaum, H. C., Wong, B. K., Schmitt, C., Nogueira-Filho, G. (2014). "Is keratinized mucosa indispensable to maintain peri-implant health? A systematic review of the literature" *J Biomed Mater Res B Appl Biomater* 102 (3). 643-50.

[41] Gobbato, L., Avila-Ortiz, G., Sohrabi, K., Wang, C. W., Karimbux, N. (2013). "The effect of keratinized mucosa width on peri-implant health: a systematic review" *Int J Oral Maxillofac Implants* 28 (6). 1536-45.

[42] Giannobile, W. V., Jung, R. E., Schwarz, F., Groups of the 2nd Osteology Foundation Consensus, Meeting. (2018). "Evidence-based knowledge on the aesthetics and maintenance of peri-implant soft tissues: Osteology Foundation Consensus Report Part 1-Effects of soft tissue augmentation procedures on the maintenance of peri-implant soft tissue health" *Clin Oral Implants Res* 29 Suppl 15 7-10.

[43] Zucchelli, G., Tavelli, L., McGuire, M. K., Rasperini, G., Feinberg, S. E., Wang, H. L., Giannobile, W. V. (2019). "Autogenous soft tissue grafting for periodontal and peri-implant plastic surgical reconstruction" *J Periodontol.*

[44] Zucchelli, G., Mele, M., Stefanini, M., Mazzotti, C., Marzadori, M., Montebugnoli, L., de Sanctis, M. (2010). "Patient morbidity and root coverage outcome after subepithelial connective tissue and de-epithelialized grafts: a comparative randomized-controlled clinical trial" *J Clin Periodontol* 37 (8). 728-38.

[45] Stefanini, M., Zucchelli, G., Marzadori, M., de Sanctis, M. (2018). "Coronally Advanced Flap with Site-Specific Application of Connective Tissue Graft for the Treatment of Multiple Adjacent Gingival Recessions: A 3-Year Follow-Up Case Series" *Int J Periodontics Restorative Dent* 38 (1). 25-33.

[46] Zeltner, M., Jung, R. E., Hammerle, C. H., Husler, J., Thoma, D. S. (2017). "Randomized controlled clinical study comparing a volume-stable collagen matrix to autogenous connective tissue grafts for soft tissue augmentation at implant sites: linear volumetric soft tissue changes up to 3 months" *J Clin Periodontol* 44 (4). 446-453.

[47] Tonetti, M. S., Cortellini, P., Pellegrini, G., Nieri, M., Bonaccini, D., Allegri, M., Bouchard, P., Cairo, F., Conforti, G., Fourmousis, I., Graziani, F., Guerrero, A., Halben, J., Malet, J., Rasperini, G., Topoll, H., Wachtel, H., Wallkamm, B., Zabalegui, I., Zuhr, O. (2018). "Xenogenic collagen matrix or autologous connective tissue graft as adjunct to coronally advanced flaps for coverage of multiple adjacent gingival recession: Randomized trial assessing non-inferiority in root coverage and superiority in oral health-related quality of life" *J Clin Periodontol* 45 (1). 78-88.

[48] Frizzera, F., de Freitas, R. M., Munoz-Chavez, O. F., Cabral, G., Shibli, J. A., Marcantonio, E., Jr. (2019). "Impact of Soft Tissue Grafts to Reduce Peri-implant Alterations After Immediate Implant Placement and Provisionalization in Compromised Sockets" *Int J Periodontics Restorative Dent* 39 (3). 381-389.

[49] Zuiderveld, E. G., Meijer, H. J. A., den Hartog, L., Vissink, A., Raghoebar, G. M. (2018). "Effect of connective tissue grafting on peri-implant tissue in single immediate implant sites: A RCT" *J Clin Periodontol* 45 (2). 253-264.

[50] Mazzotti, C., Stefanini, M., Felice, P., Bentivogli, V., Mounssif, I., Zucchelli, G. (2018). "Soft-tissue dehiscence coverage at peri-implant sites" *Periodontol 2000* 77 (1). 256-272.

[51] Zucchelli, G., Felice, P., Mazzotti, C., Marzadori, M., Mounssif, I., Monaco, C., Stefanini, M. (2018). "5-year outcomes after coverage of soft tissue dehiscence around single implants: A prospective cohort study" *Eur J Oral Implantol* 11 (2). 215-224.

[52] Hurzeler, M. B., Weng, D. (1999). "A single-incision technique to harvest subepithelial connective tissue grafts from the palate" *Int J Periodontics Restorative Dent* 19 (3). 279-87.

[53] Liu, C. L., Weisgold, A. S. (2002). "Connective tissue graft: a classification for incision design from the palatal site and clinical case reports" *Int J Periodontics Restorative Dent* 22 (4). 373-9.

[54] Lorenzana, E. R., Allen, E. P. (2000). "The single-incision palatal harvest technique: a strategy for esthetics and patient comfort" *Int J Periodontics Restorative Dent* 20 (3). 297-305.

[55] Kumar, A., Sood, V., Masamatti, S. S., Triveni, M. G., Mehta, D. S., Khatri, M., Agarwal, V. (2013). "Modified single incision technique to harvest subepithelial connective tissue graft" *J Indian Soc Periodontol* 17 (5). 676-80.

[56] Pandit, N., Khasa, M., Gugnani, S., Malik, R., Bali, D. (2016). "Comparison of two techniques of harvesting connective tissue and its effects on healing pattern at palate and recession coverage at recipient site" *Contemp Clin Dent* 7 (1). 3-10.

[57] Puri, K., Kumar, A., Khatri, M., Bansal, M., Rehan, M., Siddeshappa, S. T. (2019). "44-year journey of palatal connective tissue graft harvest: A narrative review" *J Indian Soc Periodontol* 23 (5). 395-408.

[58] Tavelli, L., Ravida, A., Lin, G. H., Del Amo, F. S., Tattan, M., Wang, H. L. (2019). "Comparison between Subepithelial Connective Tissue Graft and De-epithelialized Gingival Graft: A systematic review and a meta-analysis" *J Int Acad Periodontol* 21 (2). 82-96.

[59] Zuhr, O., Baumer, D., Hurzeler, M. (2014). "The addition of soft tissue replacement grafts in plastic periodontal and implant surgery: critical elements in design and execution" *J Clin Periodontol* 41 Suppl 15 S123-42.

[60] Jung, U. W., Um, Y. J., Choi, S. H. (2008). "Histologic observation of soft tissue acquired from maxillary tuberosity area for root coverage" *J Periodontol* 79 (5). 934-40.

[61] Zucchelli, G., Amore, C., Sforza, N. M., Montebugnoli, L., De Sanctis, M. (2003). "Bilaminar techniques for the treatment of recession-type defects. A comparative clinical study" *J Clin Periodontol* 30 (10). 862-70.

[62] Hirsch, A., Attal, U., Chai, E., Goultschin, J., Boyan, B. D., Schwartz, Z. (2001). "Root coverage and pocket reduction as combined surgical procedures" *J Periodontol* 72 (11). 1572-9.

[63] Rojo, E., Stroppa, G., Sanz-Martin, I., Gonzalez-Martin, O., Alemany, A. S., Nart, J. (2018). "Soft tissue volume gain around dental implants using autogenous subepithelial connective tissue grafts harvested from the lateral palate or tuberosity area. A randomized controlled clinical study" *J Clin Periodontol* 45 (4). 495-503.

[64] Harris, R. J. (2003). "Histologic evaluation of connective tissue grafts in humans" *Int J Periodontics Restorative Dent* 23 (6). 575-83.

[65] Sculean, A., Gruber, R., Bosshardt, D. D. (2014). "Soft tissue wound healing around teeth and dental implants" *J Clin Periodontol* 41 Suppl 15 S6-22.

[66] McGuire, M. K., Scheyer, E. T., Gwaltney, C. (2014). "Commentary: incorporating patient-reported outcomes in periodontal clinical trials" *J Periodontol* 85 (10). 1313-9.

[67] Karthikeyan, B. V., Khanna, D., Chowdhary, K. Y., Prabhuji, M. L. (2016). "The versatile subepithelial connective tissue graft: a literature update" *Gen Dent* 64 (6). e28-e33.

[68] Lektemur Alpan, A., Torumtay Cin, G. (2019). "PRF improves wound healing and postoperative discomfort after harvesting subepithelial connective tissue graft from palate: a randomized controlled trial" *Clin Oral Investig*.

[69] Stavropoulou, C., Atout, R. N., Brownlee, M., Schroth, R. J., Kelekis-Cholakis, A. (2019). "A randomized clinical trial of cyanoacrylate tissue adhesives in donor site of connective tissue grafts" *J Periodontol* 90 (6). 608-615.

[70] Brasher, W. J., Rees, T. D., Boyce, W. A. (1975). "Complications of free grafts of masticatory mucosa" *J Periodontol* 46 (3). 133-8.

[71] Reiser, G. M., Bruno, J. F., Mahan, P. E., Larkin, L. H. (1996). "The subepithelial connective tissue graft palatal donor site: anatomic considerations for surgeons" *Int J Periodontics Restorative Dent* 16 (2). 130-7.

[72] Monnet-Corti, V., Santini, A., Glise, J. M., Fouque-Deruelle, C., Dillier, F. L., Liebart, M. F., Borghetti, A. (2006). "Connective tissue graft for gingival recession treatment: assessment of the maximum graft dimensions at the palatal vault as a donor site" *J Periodontol* 77 (5). 899-902.

[73] Tavelli, L., Barootchi, S., Ravida, A., Oh, T. J., Wang, H. L. (2019). "What Is the Safety Zone for Palatal Soft Tissue Graft Harvesting Based on the Locations of the Greater Palatine Artery and Foramen? A Systematic Review" *J Oral Maxillofac Surg* 77 (2). 271 e1-271 e9.

INDEX

A

acid, 22, 36, 37, 38, 102, 115
adaptation, viii, 2, 116, 122
adipose, 3, 4, 5, 10, 71, 96, 100, 128
adipose tissue, 4, 5, 10, 96, 128
aesthetics, 102, 104, 105, 108, 115, 131, 136
alveolar macrophage, 5
alveolar ridge, 81, 114
anti-inflammatory agents, 19
anti-inflammatory drugs, 20
autoantibodies, 50
autogenous grafts, 114
autografts, 112, 114
autoimmune disease, 50
autosomal dominant, 45, 46, 47, 48

B

basal lamina, 15, 16
basal layer, 74
basement membrane, 15, 33, 34, 35, 46, 47
biochemistry, 13
biosynthesis, 28, 37
bleeding, 63, 73, 75, 78, 100, 101, 102, 122, 126, 130
blood, vii, 1, 3, 5, 6, 7, 9, 10, 15, 16, 21, 33, 48, 49, 53, 56, 58, 63, 65, 73, 78, 79, 80, 96, 97, 98, 100, 101, 103, 104, 106, 112, 118, 126
blood circulation, 6
blood supply, 53, 56, 58, 63, 65, 78, 79, 96, 97, 98, 100, 101, 103, 104, 112, 118, 126
blood vessels, 5, 15, 16, 21, 33, 49, 73, 106
bloodstream, viii, 2
bone, vii, 1, 4, 12, 14, 16, 17, 18, 21, 33, 34, 39, 43, 44, 61, 62, 63, 66, 73, 76, 81, 95, 98, 99, 102, 107, 114, 115, 116, 118, 121, 122, 123, 124, 127, 128, 129
bone cells, viii, 2
bone marrow, vii, 1, 12
brain, 3

C

capillary, 11, 15, 16, 51
carbon, 6, 9, 35
carbon dioxide, 9

carboxyl, 35, 36, 37
carboxylic acid, 36
cartilage, vii, 1, 4, 8, 9, 17, 21, 28, 33, 34, 41, 46
cell differentiation, 21
cell division, 8
cell surface, 16
central nervous system, 3, 5
chondroitin sulfate, 9, 17, 115
chromosome, 48
circulation, 3, 9, 55, 65, 106
closure, 55, 56, 58, 67, 77, 98, 99, 101, 125, 126
collagen, vii, 1, 3, 9, 10, 11, 13, 14, 15, 16, 18, 19, 20, 21, 22, 23, 24, 25, 27, 28, 29, 30, 31, 32, 33, 34, 35, 36, 37, 38, 39, 40, 41, 42, 43, 44, 45, 46, 47, 48, 49, 50, 104, 115, 136
complications, vii, ix, 20, 48, 77, 80, 107, 113, 115, 129, 130
composition, 13, 14, 28, 33, 34, 37
compression, 69, 70, 99, 100
connective tissue, vii, viii, ix, 1, 2, 3, 4, 5, 7, 8, 9, 10, 11, 12, 13, 14, 15, 16, 17, 18, 19, 20, 21, 24, 33, 34, 43, 45, 48, 49, 51, 52, 53, 54, 55, 58, 61, 62, 64, 67, 69, 70, 72, 73, 74, 75, 76, 78, 79, 81, 93, 94, 95, 96, 97, 99, 100, 101, 103, 104, 105, 106, 107, 108, 109, 110, 111, 113, 114, 115, 118, 123, 124, 125, 126, 127, 128, 131, 132, 133, 134, 135, 136, 137, 138, 139
contraceptives, 19
control group, 129
cytoplasm, 5, 7, 24, 30, 41
cytoskeleton, 12

D

defects, ix, 43, 45, 46, 52, 68, 70, 78, 79, 80, 81, 93, 97, 103, 104, 105, 107, 108, 109, 111, 114, 116, 118, 120, 122, 129, 132, 133, 134, 138
defense mechanisms, 3
deficiencies, 81, 122, 129
deficiency, 50, 118
dehiscence, 122, 137
dental implants, 114, 129, 135, 138
dental plaque, 19
dentist, 17
depth, 60, 78, 95, 103, 114, 116, 122
derivatives, 24, 37
dermis, vii, 1, 11, 12, 33
discomfort, 56, 76, 80, 97, 107, 119, 129, 139
diseases, 13, 43, 44, 45, 46
disorder, 47, 48, 49
displacement, 51
distribution, viii, 2, 13, 14, 46

E

ecchymosis, 80, 107, 129
Ehlers-Danlos syndrome, 44, 45, 46
elastin, 9, 11, 16
electron, 7, 39, 40
electron microscopy, 7, 39
enamel, 55, 102, 114, 118, 133, 134
environmental factors, 43
enzyme, 41, 43, 46
enzymes, 6, 29, 41, 42, 44
epidermolysis bullosa, 47, 48
epiglottis, 9
epithelia, 3, 109
epithelium, 15, 16, 35, 47, 58, 60, 61, 64, 69, 74, 75, 94, 95, 98, 99, 100, 105, 106, 107, 115, 123, 126, 128
erythrocytes, viii, 2
esophagus, 20, 50
estrogen, 18
ethylene, 102
evidence, 116

Index

evolution, 12
execution, 108, 109, 138
exons, 40, 45
exposure, 96, 110
extracellular matrix, 3, 8, 12, 16, 18, 19, 24, 31, 50, 132

F

fibers, vii, 1, 3, 8, 9, 10, 11, 14, 15, 16, 21, 22, 24, 30, 50, 115, 128
fibroblast proliferation, 18
fibroblasts, viii, 2, 3, 5, 9, 12, 16, 18, 19, 24, 28, 49, 115
fibrosis, 12, 27, 49, 50
fibrous tissue, vii, 1, 4
first molar, 70, 72, 96, 100, 128, 130
formation, 16, 18, 22, 24, 25, 27, 37, 39, 43, 48, 56, 67, 80, 100, 102

G

gastrointestinal tract, 20
genes, 40, 41, 44, 45, 47, 48
gingival, viii, ix, 2, 15, 16, 18, 19, 20, 51, 52, 53, 54, 55, 58, 62, 63, 64, 69, 70, 72, 73, 77, 78, 79, 80, 81, 93, 94, 96, 97, 98, 99, 100, 102, 105, 107, 110, 111, 112, 113, 114, 116, 117, 120, 121, 123, 125, 126, 127, 128, 129, 131, 132, 133, 134, 135, 136, 139
gingival epithelium, viii, 2
gingival overgrowth, 19
gingival pigmentation, 79, 97
gingival recession, viii, ix, 51, 52, 53, 54, 70, 73, 77, 81, 89, 93, 94, 95, 96, 110, 111, 112, 113, 114, 116, 117, 120, 121, 123, 128, 131, 132, 133, 134, 135, 136, 139
glycine, 22, 35, 37, 38, 39, 40, 44, 45, 46
glycoproteins, 3, 11, 17, 115

glycosaminoglycans, 15
graft technique, 58, 95, 109, 110, 126
growth, 8, 17, 18, 27, 46, 132
growth factor, 18, 132

H

harvesting, vii, viii, ix, 53, 55, 67, 69, 73, 76, 81, 93, 94, 95, 96, 98, 108, 110, 111, 113, 114, 123, 126, 127, 130, 131, 137, 139
healing, ix, 4, 18, 21, 24, 27, 51, 54, 56, 60, 61, 63, 65, 67, 75, 76, 80, 81, 83, 84, 93, 94, 97, 98, 99, 103, 105, 106, 107, 110, 112, 119, 121, 122, 125, 126, 127, 129, 133, 137, 138, 139
health, 52, 121, 122, 135, 136
hearing loss, 44, 47
heart valves, 49
heat shock protein, 43
height, 81, 107, 114, 129
helical conformation, 22, 38
human, vii, 1, 3, 14, 108, 109, 111
human body, vii, 1, 3, 14
hydroxyapatite, 111
hydroxyl, 35, 37
hygiene, 51
hypersensitivity, 51
hypertension, 47

I

immune response, 4, 6
immunoglobulin, 7
immunomodulatory, 105
implant placement, 122
implantology, 114
implants, 97, 101, 114, 116, 128, 135, 137
incisor, 60, 120, 121
individuals, 47, 50
infection, 6, 80, 107, 129

inflammation, 17, 78, 114, 122
inflammatory disease, 13
integration, 58, 95, 106
integrity, 24, 47, 126
interface, 6, 15, 105

L

lesions, 19, 49, 133
leukocytes, viii, 2
ligament, 12, 14, 16, 21, 27, 33, 51
light, ix, 6, 7, 38, 40, 44, 113
lysine, 22, 29, 35, 37, 39, 42, 50

M

macrophages, viii, 2, 3, 4, 6
management, 79, 81
manipulation, 99, 127
medical, 17, 18
medical history, 17
medication, 17
melting temperature, 42
membrane permeability, 20
membranes, 3, 31, 105
mesenchymal stem cells, 111
mesenchyme, 2, 11, 81
meta-analysis, 126, 134, 135, 138
modifications, 25, 43, 53
molecular mass, 42
molecules, 2, 13, 22, 23, 25, 28, 29, 30, 39, 40, 42, 43, 44, 45, 50
morbidity, 61, 75, 76, 99, 129, 136
mucosa, viii, 2, 16, 33, 49, 50, 53, 59, 61, 65, 71, 74, 77, 94, 95, 100, 101, 104, 106, 109, 114, 116, 122, 135, 139
mucous membrane, viii, 2, 48
mutations, 44, 45, 46, 47, 48
myofibroblasts, 12, 24

N

necrosis, 75, 77, 101, 106, 107, 129
nervous system, 3, 48
nucleus, 5, 7, 24, 30, 43

O

oral cavity, viii, 2, 20
oral health, 50, 136
organ, 3, 12, 17, 47
organelles, 7
organic solvents, 5
organs, 3, 4, 9, 11, 31, 33, 49
osteoarthritis, 20, 47
osteogenesis imperfecta, 44, 45

P

pain, 20, 49, 65, 107, 118, 129
palate, viii, ix, 2, 52, 53, 58, 59, 61, 62, 64, 70, 71, 72, 80, 95, 96, 98, 99, 100, 102, 104, 107, 110, 113, 114, 128, 129, 130, 137, 138, 139
perforation, 71, 72, 77, 100, 101
peri-implant soft tissue, 114, 121, 122, 133, 136
periodontal, v, ix, 1, 12, 13, 14, 15, 16, 17, 18, 20, 21, 27, 46, 47, 49, 51, 52, 58, 61, 63, 72, 74, 81, 82, 85, 87, 88, 89, 91, 92, 94, 100, 108, 109, 112, 113, 114, 115, 116, 127, 131, 132, 133, 134, 136, 138, 139
periodontal disease, 20, 49
periodontal involvement, 46
periodontal plastic surgery, ix, 94, 108, 113, 114, 116, 131, 132, 134
periodontist, 51
periosteum, 62, 65, 66, 67, 69, 76, 95, 100, 102, 107, 111, 115, 127, 128

Index

phagocytic cells, viii, 2, 5
plastic surgery, 114
polypeptide, 22, 23, 25, 36, 37, 38, 41
predictability, 54, 80, 95, 97, 101, 102
progenitor cells, 12
progesterone, 18
pro-inflammatory, 6
proliferation, 21
proline, 22, 23, 29, 35, 36, 37, 38, 39, 50
promoter, 40, 41
prosthesis, 78, 119
proteins, viii, 2, 11, 12, 13, 14, 16, 21, 28, 30, 31, 36, 48
proteoglycans, 3, 11, 13, 14, 15, 16, 20, 40, 115

R

reactions, 6, 12, 30, 41, 50
receptors, 16, 17, 18
recession, viii, ix, 51, 52, 53, 59, 60, 61, 63, 66, 68, 70, 73, 77, 78, 81, 93, 94, 95, 96, 103, 104, 109, 110, 113, 114, 116, 117, 118, 120, 121, 122, 123, 131, 132, 133, 134, 135, 136, 137, 138, 139
reconstruction, 52, 78, 79, 97, 114, 136
red blood cells, viii, 2
regeneration, 13, 52, 94, 109, 111, 116, 131, 133
regenerative capacity, 13
repair, 24, 27, 66, 100, 112, 115, 116
residues, 23, 37, 38, 41, 42, 43
reticulum, 7, 23, 24, 25, 28, 41
risk, 65, 96, 114, 124, 126, 130
root, viii, 48, 51, 52, 53, 54, 55, 59, 60, 67, 70, 80, 93, 94, 96, 97, 101, 102, 103, 104, 107, 108, 109, 110, 114, 116, 117, 119, 126, 129, 132, 133, 134, 136, 138

S

skin, 2, 12, 21, 33, 45, 48, 49
smooth muscle, 12
soft tissue grafting, 114, 134, 136
species, 14, 16, 17, 34
squamous cell carcinoma, 12
stability, 23, 53, 54, 116, 121, 134, 135
structural gene, 44
structural protein, 20, 21
structure, viii, 2, 3, 13, 21, 22, 34, 38, 39, 40, 43, 101, 115
subepithelial basement membrane, 16
subepithelial connective tissue, v, vii, ix, 52, 53, 54, 75, 79, 80, 81, 83, 84, 86, 87, 89, 91, 92, 94, 95, 105, 107, 108, 109, 110, 111, 113, 114, 115, 132, 133, 134, 135, 136, 137, 138, 139
subepithelial connective tissue graft, vii, ix, 52, 53, 54, 75, 79, 80, 81, 83, 84, 86, 87, 89, 91, 94, 105, 107, 108, 109, 110, 111, 113, 132, 133, 134, 135, 137, 138, 139
submucosa, 50, 52, 71, 95, 102, 128
surgical technique, 52, 115
suture, 53, 64, 65, 69, 80, 96, 103, 107, 127, 129
synthesis, 18, 23, 27, 28, 36, 41, 42, 50

T

techniques, vii, ix, 52, 53, 75, 81, 93, 94, 97, 98, 101, 108, 111, 113, 114, 116, 126, 127, 129, 131, 135, 137, 138
teeth, viii, 2, 21, 28, 44, 46, 51, 52, 55, 58, 63, 64, 66, 73, 74, 78, 81, 95, 98, 99, 103, 114, 116, 123, 124, 127, 128, 131, 134, 138
tissue, vii, viii, 1, 2, 3, 4, 5, 6, 8, 9, 10, 11, 13, 15, 16, 19, 20, 21, 24, 27, 28, 34, 35, 39, 40, 41, 42, 44, 48, 51, 52, 53, 54, 55, 58, 59, 60, 61, 62, 63, 64, 65, 66, 67, 68,

69, 71, 72, 73, 74, 76, 78, 79, 80, 81, 93, 94, 95, 96, 97, 99, 100, 102, 103, 104, 105, 106, 107, 108, 109, 110, 111, 112, 114, 115, 116, 118, 119, 121, 122, 123, 124, 125, 126, 127, 128, 129, 130, 131, 132, 133, 134, 135, 136, 137, 138, 139
treatment, 17, 20, 52, 53, 54, 81, 94, 108, 111, 114, 116, 117, 118, 119, 131, 132, 133, 134, 138, 139
trial, 116, 118, 132, 133, 134, 135, 136, 139
tumor progression, 12

V

vessels, 71, 96, 106, 115, 128, 130

W

white blood cells, viii, 2, 3
wound healing, 4, 18, 24, 51, 110, 127, 138, 139